SCOTLAND HEALTH DEFICIT: AN EXPLANATION AND A PLAN

Oliver Gillie

Scotland has an extreme climate characterised by very little sunshine. Its people have low levels of vitamin D because most vitamin D comes from the effect of sun on skin. Scots also have high levels of chronic illness – among the highest in the world. Low levels of vitamin D are now known to be an important cause of chronic illness including cancer and heart disease. But vitamin D has received little or no attention from policy makers in Scotland.

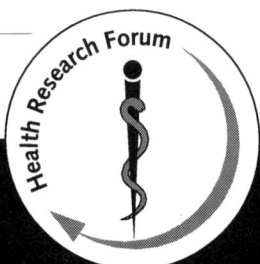

Published by Health Research Forum, 68 Whitehall Park, London N19 3TN

email: olivergillie@blueyonder.co.uk phone: +4420 7561 9677

First edition 2008

Health Research Forum Publishing

Health Research Forum is a private non-profit making research organisation founded by Oliver Gillie in 2004.

ISBN numbers: 9553200-2-X and 978-0-9553200-2-6

Disclosure

Oliver Gillie has received no personal remuneration from commercial interests that might profit from any aspect of this work. In particular he has never accepted personal payments from makers of sunlamps or vitamin supplements, or their proxies.

Key words:
Scotland, Scottish effect, mortality, chronic disease, vitamin D, deficiency, sunlight, sunlamps, sunbeds, tanning, UVB, climate, cancer, heart disease, heart failure, hypertension, blood pressure, stroke, bone disease, rickets, osteomalacia, osteoporosis, multiple sclerosis, diabetes, Crohn's disease, rheumatoid arthritis, asthma, autoimmune disease, chest infection, tuberculosis, back pain, muscle strength, sport, fitness, stress fracture, tooth decay, public health, health policy, SunSmart, Cancer Research UK, sunbathing, melanoma, skin cancer, nutrition, breast feeding, Orkney, Shetland, Faroes, Iceland, multiple sclerosis epidemic, childhood leukaemia (leukemia) epidemic, fish diet, Sir Richard Doll, James Watson.

Contact: Oliver Gillie, 68 Whitehall Park, London N19 3TN
email: olivergillie@blueyonder.co.uk phone: +4420 7561 9677

Design and production: Design Unlimited
Editing and sub-editing: Jim Anderson and Michael Crozier

Scotland's health deficit – an explanation and a plan
is highly recommended by international experts. This is what they said:

"This impressive piece of work has major significance for Scotland's health. Dr Gillie's meticulous research and careful argument call for serious attention from its policy makers."
Professor Joy Townsend, London School of Hygiene and Tropical Medicine

"Oliver Gillie makes a very compelling case that widespread vitamin D deficiency contributes importantly to the many health problems that plague Scotland."
Edward Giovannucci, Professor of Nutrition and Epidemiology, Department of Nutrition, Harvard School of Public Health

"A collaboration of researchers in Scotland have been inspired to think again about the potential role of vitamin D in improving Scotland's health. It is a privilege to be working with Dr Oliver Gillie who has a long-standing interest in Scotland, its people and vitamin D, as is clear from a reading of this book."
Dr Raj Bhopal, Bruce and John Usher Professor of Public Health, University of Edinburgh

"I found your book very interesting. I grew up in Scotland, and I often recall my mother, on rare sunny days, exhorting me to go out and 'soak up the sun', as it was good for me. I'm sure she was passing on an 'old wives' remedy with real substance. I really think we need to find a way to undo the short-sightedness of the broad public health campaigns that try to stop entire populations from being out in the sun 'unprotected'."
Dr Colin Begg, Memorial Sloan-Kettering Cancer Centre, New York

"The UK has it bad, but Scotland has it even worse when it comes to a lack of sunshine. It is all too easy to be sceptical that a technology so simple as vitamin D could play a major role in correcting a breadth of health deficits. Oliver Gillie has laid out out the problems and the solutions so logically that only the most incurable sceptic could remain unswayed."
Dr Reinhold Vieth, Professor, Department of Nutritional Sciences, University of Toronto

"Gillie has collated a large body of data from different diseases and makes a strong case for the role of vitamin D deficiency in the pathogenesis of a variety of disorders ranging from heart disease to autoimmunity. There is no source that covers this so comprehensively and after reading this monograph more questions will and should be asked about the public policies that have continued the same practices now for half a century. There are additional scientific questions to be sure, but continued inaction at a public health level warrants urgent review. Gillie has performed an extremely important service in tirelessly promoting the ideas in this book and he has many strong scientific supporters. I include myself among these, and the evidence suggests that at least some of the diseases he reviews will have vitamin D as their basis. At the very least we need an urgent policy rethink and need to ensure that the *status quo* is not inertial in nature."
George Ebers, Action Research Professor of Clinical Neurology, Oxford University, England

"Nearly a century ago it became obvious that vitamin D can cure rickets in infants, an illness also known as English disease. Oliver Gillie shows us that vitamin D deficiency is still frequent in the adult English population and is even more frequent in Scots. This situation presumably contributes to many chronic diseases. Hopefully, the present book opens the eyes of many health authorities that a century after vitamin D's discovery its deficiency has not been erased yet."
Dr Armin Zittermann, Department of Cardio-Thoracic Surgery, Ruhr University Bochum, Bad Oeynhausen, Germany

"I visited Scotland in 2004 at the request of Dr George Ebers to discuss the role of vitamin D and multiple sclerosis with Scottish neurologists. I returned for a holiday three years later, went into a chemist and found that vitamin tablets still contained only 200 IU of vitamin D, a woeful amount. Hopefully this wonderful piece of work by Dr Gillie will change the *status quo*."
Dr Bruce W. Hollis, Professor, Medical University of South Carolina, Charleston, South Carolina

"Oliver Gillie has an established track record in the presentation of scientific material in an informative and balanced way and is exceptionally well informed about vitamin D. His report on the 'Scottish paradox' details evidence suggesting that simple measures to correct lack of vitamin D, so common in Scotland, would contribute substantially to reducing the burden of chronic disorders such as diabetes and heart disease.

"I have vivid memories of my childhood in Troon where herrings, cabbage, oatmeal and cod liver oil were common in our diet. Now many years later I am grateful for good health that probably owes something to those nourishing staples, despite little enough sunshine in those early years.

"I am in no doubt that the bodies concerned with public health in Scotland will find this report useful in devising cost-effective measures for avoiding hypovitaminosis D and thereby reducing the burden of chronic disease on the Scottish people, on the health service and the national budget."
Dr Barbara Boucher, honorary senior lecturer, Centre for Diabetes and Metabolic Medicine, Barts and the London Medical and Dental School, London

"Dr Gillie's book is both timely and enlightening. There is a mountain of new scientific literature that supports the concept that vitamin D deficiency may be responsible for increased risk of many chronic diseases including cancer, heart disease, diabetes and infectious diseases. Vitamin D deficiency has become a world-wide health problem and is very evident in Scotland. Dr. Gillie provides a lucid review of the evidence linking chronic vitamin D deficiency to many health problems that particularly plague the Scots. Sensible sun exposure, that is when the sun is shining in Scotland, along with a very aggressive program to implement vitamin D food fortification is greatly needed, and the recommendations made by Dr Gillie are insightful and should be implemented immediately."
Dr Michael Holick, Department of Medicine, Boston University Medical Center, Boston, USA

In remembrance of my father John Calder Gillie, nautical instrument maker, optician, and Quaker philanthropist

For my wife, Jan Thompson, and my two sons, Calder and Sholto, who have encouraged me to continue with this project

Acknowledgements and thanks

I could never have undertaken this work without the help of very many people who have freely discussed their research with me and taken the trouble to explain details to me. I am greatly indebted to them for their unstinting help.

To the best of my knowledge the hypothesis advanced here, that the deficit in health of Scots compared with English people and other Europeans can be accounted for by low sunlight levels and insufficient vitamin D, has not been stated explicitly before, or not in any detail. However this hypothesis and the conclusions in this book rest on the work of very many others who have shown the way with their studies of Scottish health, vitamin D and sunlight. Without their patient and painstaking research over many years this hypothesis could not have been developed.

In particular the works of Phil Hanlon and colleagues on the "Scottish effect", and of Richard Mitchell and colleagues on unexplained high levels of heart disease in Scotland deserve great credit for identifying the problem. While the work of RW Morris, PH Whincup, and AG Shaper and others at the British Regional Heart Survey on the geographic variation in heart disease in Britain has also been very important. Jonathan Elford and colleagues' studies of place of birth and migration in connection with heart disease have provided further important insights. These studies and many others credited within have been most important in developing an understanding of health in Scotland, of the "Scottish effect" and of vitamin D insufficiency.

I also wish to acknowledge the dedicated pioneering work of many scientists over many years to demonstrate the vital role of vitamin D in human life. Among these pioneers I must mention Reinhold Vieth, Michael Holick, Bill Grant, Bruce Hollis, Robert Heaney, John Cannell, the Garland brothers and their colleagues, George Ebers and colleagues, Barbara Boucher, Elina Hypponen, Adrian Martineau and many others. Any list of this kind does an injustice to others by leaving them out. Please allow me to thank all those whose important work is mentioned in the text but whose names are not mentioned here.

Finally I am also specially grateful to my wife and family who have encouraged and supported me in undertaking this work, to Michael Crozier and Jim Anderson for their practical help and encouragement, to Joy Townsend for her detailed comments and guidance, and to Julian Peto for his friendship and wisdom.

Oliver Gillie
April 2008

Contents

Summary

People living in Scotland have a lower average level of vitamin D in their bodies than people in England and a higher incidence of several common chronic diseases. The difference in vitamin D levels is a result of Scotland's northerly location, which allows less opportunity for exposure of the skin to sunlight. A healthy person in Europe or North America obtains more than 90% of their vitamin D by exposure of skin to the sun. The low levels of vitamin D in the Scottish population can explain, at least in part, the higher levels of certain chronic diseases and the higher death rates found in Scotland compared to England and most other Western European countries.

While health has been improving in Scotland, the advance is not as fast as in other European countries, and at the present rate Scotland will never catch up. This report calls for urgent action by Scotland's government to take new measures that will give the country its best chance of improving health and of catching up with other European countries that have more favourable climates.

Insufficient vitamin D is an important factor increasing the risk or severity of several chronic diseases including several cancers, heart disease, stroke, multiple sclerosis, high blood pressure, diabetes (types 1 and 2), and arthritis as well as bone disease and fractures that frequently lead to death in old people. Most of these, and certain other ills, occur more frequently in Scotland compared with England – a difference that may be accounted for largely by the difference in available sunlight between the two countries. Looking at multiple sclerosis alone, Scotland has a higher percentage of sufferers than any other country in the world, and the second highest percentage for Crohn's disease.

However successive reports on the state of Scottish health have failed to recognise that insufficient sunlight and vitamin D are important risk factors for health in Scotland. The purpose of this book is to draw attention to this gap and show how major gains in Scottish health can be expected from relatively simple preventive measures.

Multiple sclerosis, diabetes type 1, and Crohn's disease are autoimmune diseases which have become much more common in Scotland during the last 30 years or more. It is no exaggeration to say that Scotland is in the grip of a serious epidemic of autoimmune disease. Similar increases are occurring in other countries but the epidemic appears to be more extensive in Scotland than elsewhere and may be caused in large part by insufficient vitamin D.

The vitamin D status of the Scottish population could be boosted by making supplements available cheaply and/or by fortifying food with vitamin D. A relatively small investment might reduce personal misery of very large numbers of people as well as save large sums presently spent on illness and disability in Scotland. The problem of vitamin D insufficiency requires the same urgent attention from government as smoking, alcoholism or obesity.

Vitamin D status can be improved without the personal denial or discipline needed by smokers, drinkers, or dieters who attempt to give up cigarettes, or reduce alcohol or food intake. The principal factor preventing improvement in vitamin D levels at present is lack of government action in facilitating the availability of vitamin D supplements together with lack of knowledge of the problem among health professionals and the public.

Mistaken advice from government in London and from Cancer Research UK to avoid exposure to the sun between 11am and 3pm can only have pushed down average levels of vitamin D in the past. Official advice needs to be brought up to date so that the public is encouraged to sunbathe without burning, since burning appears to be the major risk factor for skin cancer rather than sun exposure itself.

Introduction:
Scotland's health deficit

Scotland is bottom of the premier league of nations when it comes to health [1]. People in Scotland die younger on average than in almost any other Western European nation of similar stature – see figure 1 below [1]. Premature mortality in Scotland's central belt reaching from Glasgow to Edinburgh is close to that of the former East Germany (German Democratic Republic) and is the highest in Europe [2]. This position has puzzled scientists for at least a generation. In this review I offer an explanation of the Scottish health deficit and suggest how major gains in health could be obtained in Scotland by relatively simple measures.

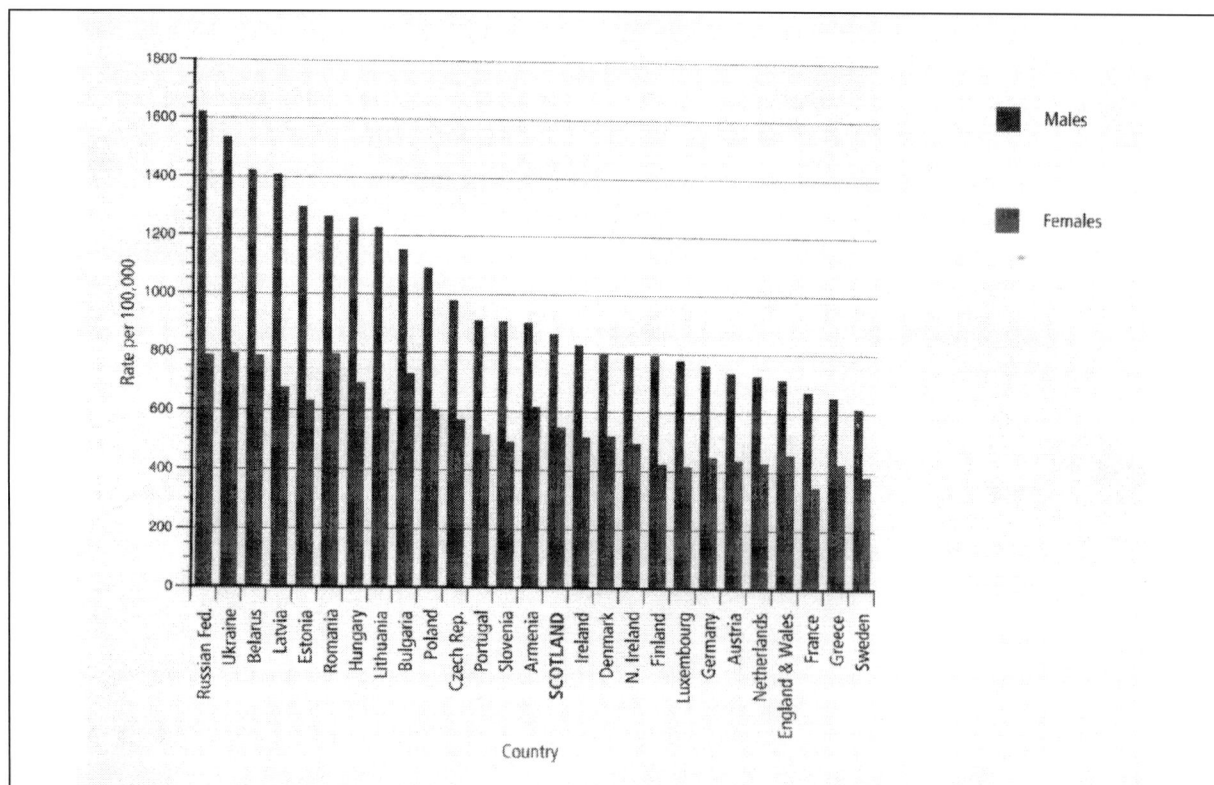

Figure 1. Comparison of all-cause mortality rates per 100,000 population (age-standardised) for males and females. Mortality of Scots females is even higher in this international league than that of Scots males. Source: WHO.

Scotland's geographical position on the edge of the Atlantic and in the most northern part of Europe gives it a cloudy maritime climate with much reduced hours of sunshine compared with other northern countries of continental Europe or with southern parts of the UK. Glasgow, because of its position on the western seacoast, gets no more sun than places above the Arctic Circle. As a result Scots people obtain much less exposure to the sun [3] and so obtain insufficient vitamin D [4-7], compared with people in England and most other European countries – see Figures 2-4. Many scientific studies have found that low levels of vitamin D are associated with higher mortality from cancer, heart disease, raised blood pressure, stroke, diabetes and other diseases [8, 9] which account for up to 70% of total mortality in Scotland and other industrial countries.

The suggestion made here that excess mortality in Scotland is the result of insufficient vitamin D is bolstered by international studies showing that people who take a vitamin D supplement live longer and are less likely to die early from cancer, heart disease or other ills [10]. Taking a regular supplement of vitamin D may reduce overall mortality by 7% or more according to a recent analysis of pooled results of international trials of vitamin D [10]. Most of these trials were originally undertaken to study prevention of osteoporosis, fractures or other conditions but tak-

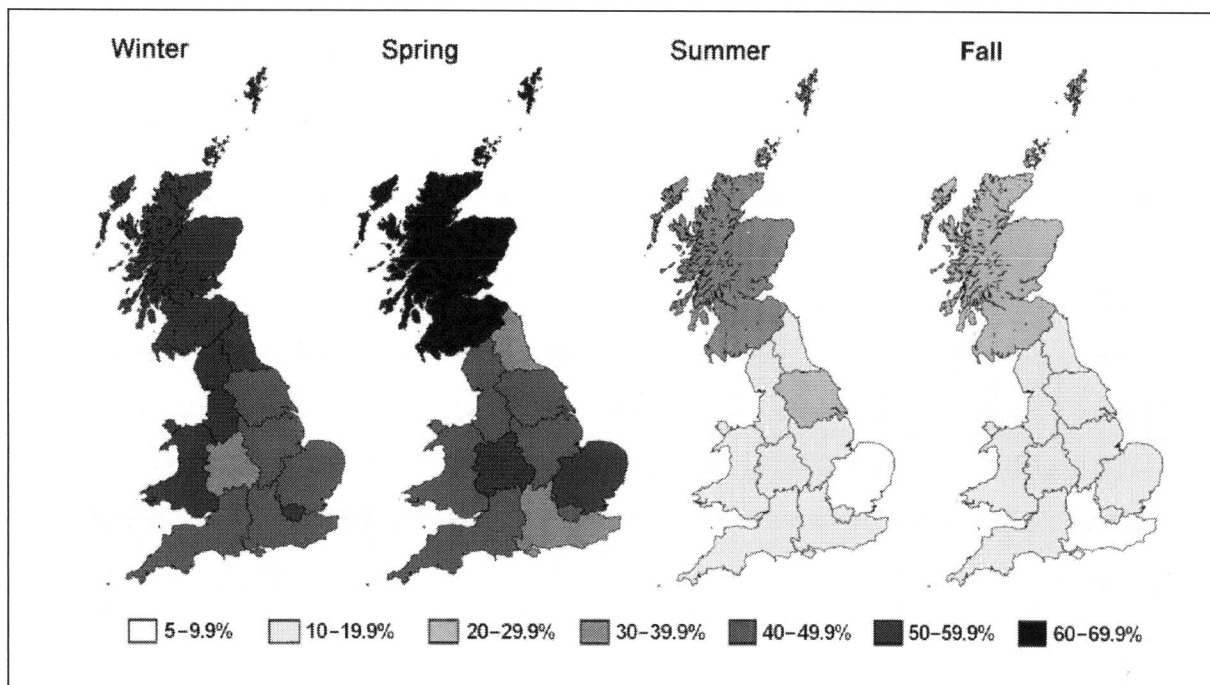

Figure 2. Seasonal and geographical variation in the prevalence of hypovitaminosis D (25-hydroxyvitamin D less than 40 nmol/L) in Great Britain. Low levels of vitamin D are particularly obvious in Scotland in summer and autumn. From *Hypponen and Power* [5].

en together they show a remarkable overall improvement in mortality of those taking a vitamin D supplement. Another study (double blind and randomised) found that 55-year-old women in Nebraska who were given a daily dose of 1100 IUs of vitamin D over a period of four years were half as likely to suffer cancer as control women given a placebo [11].

Many reasons – smoking, alcoholism, and poverty – have been considered as explanations of the excess ill health and mortality in Scotland [1]. But until now, insufficient vitamin D has not been considered as a possible explanation. Numerous reports on Scottish Health refer to problems of smoking, obesity and alcohol but make no mention of vitamin D or of the problems from too little sunshine in the Scottish climate [2, 12-17].

Health Protection Scotland, the body which is charged by the Scottish Executive with the task of strengthening and co-ordinating health protection north of the border makes no mention of vitamin D on its website although detailed information about other risk factors for disease are listed [18]. And at the time of writing the Scottish Public Health Observatory, which has a similar brief, makes no mention of vitamin D insufficiency as a risk factor for cancer, heart disease, or multiple sclerosis and does not even mention rickets, the childhood bone disease that is re-emerging in Scotland as a result of insufficient vitamin D [8, 19].

It is only in the last 10 years or so that the many functions of vitamin D essential for health, besides the regulation of calcium absorption and the growth of bone, have become known and knowledge of its importance for health is only now reaching specialists in public health [20]. Practising doctors and even nutritionists have not generally been aware of these developments until very recently. However, internationally recognised experts now acknowledge that insufficient vitamin D is a major risk factor for chronic disease comparable in importance to smoking, alcohol or obesity [20].

This review explains the relevance of new findings concerning vitamin D to the health of people in Scotland and outlines a plan to produce a "step-change" in Scottish health. Much political attention has been given to health inequalities within both Scotland and England [21]. The health inequalities between our two nations deserve equally urgent attention and urgent political action.

Chapter 1:
The "sunshine vitamin" and the Scots' climate

1. Scotland gets less sun, Scots get less D

The major population concentrations in southern England and central Scotland are only some 300 miles apart on a north-south axis. London is at latitude 51.5° north while Glasgow and Edinburgh are at 56° north. But this smal difference in distance makes a large difference to the amount of "biologically active" UV light that reaches earth and is capable of inducing the formation of vitamin D in skin.

Even in Scotland sunlight remains the major source of vitamin D. But it is only certain wavelengths of UV that induce formation of vitamin D in skin while other wavelengths are inactive. The active part of the UV spectrum lies in the range known as UVB and it is absorbed more readily in the atmosphere than other wavelengths. So when the sun is low in the sky and the light travels through a longer path in the atmosphere the active UVB component of sunlight is reduced, and when the angle of the sun is below about 45° active UVB is almost completely absent from sunlight.

Scotland receives some 30-50% less biological active UVB than much of England (see Figure 3 [3, 22]). The sun north of the border is lower in the sky for most of the year and so more of the active UVB is absorbed in the atmosphere than at lower latitudes. A definitive geographical comparison of "effective UVB", that is UVB weighted for its biological effect in reddening skin, has been made by Colin Driscoll of the National Radiological Protection Board at Chilton in Oxfordshire and others [23]. UVB that reddens the skin is often taken as much the same wavelength as the UVB that is most effective in synthesising vitamin D.

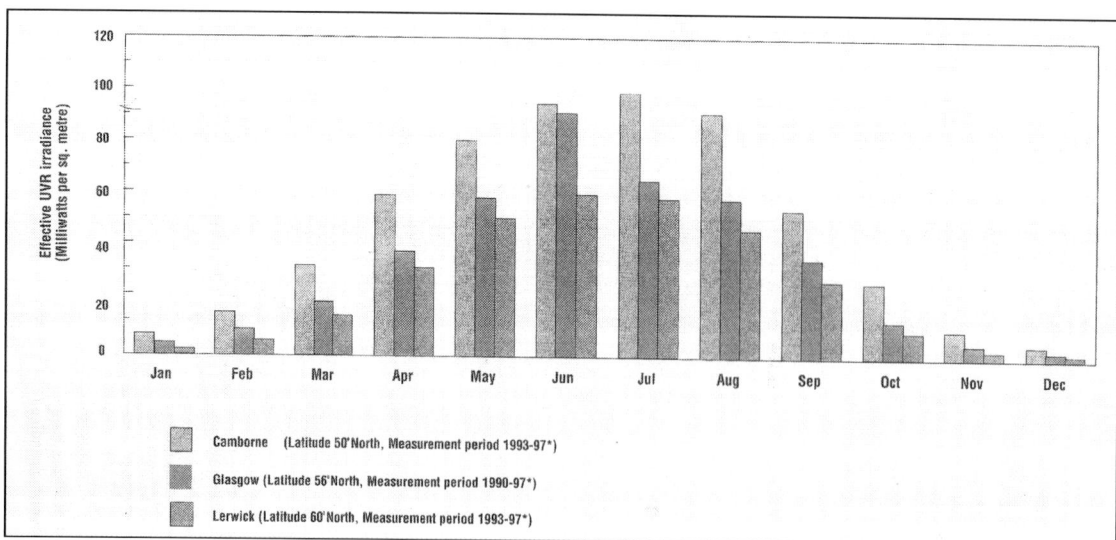

Figure 3. The North/South difference in sunlight – mean effective UV radiation (UVR) at 3 UK sites. Glasgow has substantially less sun than Camborne (SW England) in all months except June. UVR measured at 12 hrs GMT and weighted for biological effectiveness in the skin. Source: National Radiological Protection Board (unpublished data). From *Nutrition and Bone Health*, Dept of Health Report on Health and Social Subjects, No 49, Stationery Office, 1998 [3]

Driscoll's comparison shows that Glasgow obtains the same amount of UVB in the effective range as Kiruna, which is above the Arctic Circle in northern Sweden. Lund in southern Sweden is on almost the same latitude as Glasgow and obtains 50% more sun, showing the effect of cloud and overcast skies on our western coast. Durham, which is on the east coast of England and only 70 miles south of Glasgow, also obtains 50% more sun than Glasgow. This shows that there are important East/West differences in sun over the British Isles as well as the north/south differences.

However the length of the summer season and the air temperature is as important as the total amount of sunlight available in determining how much sun exposure people will get per year in a given locality. The summer

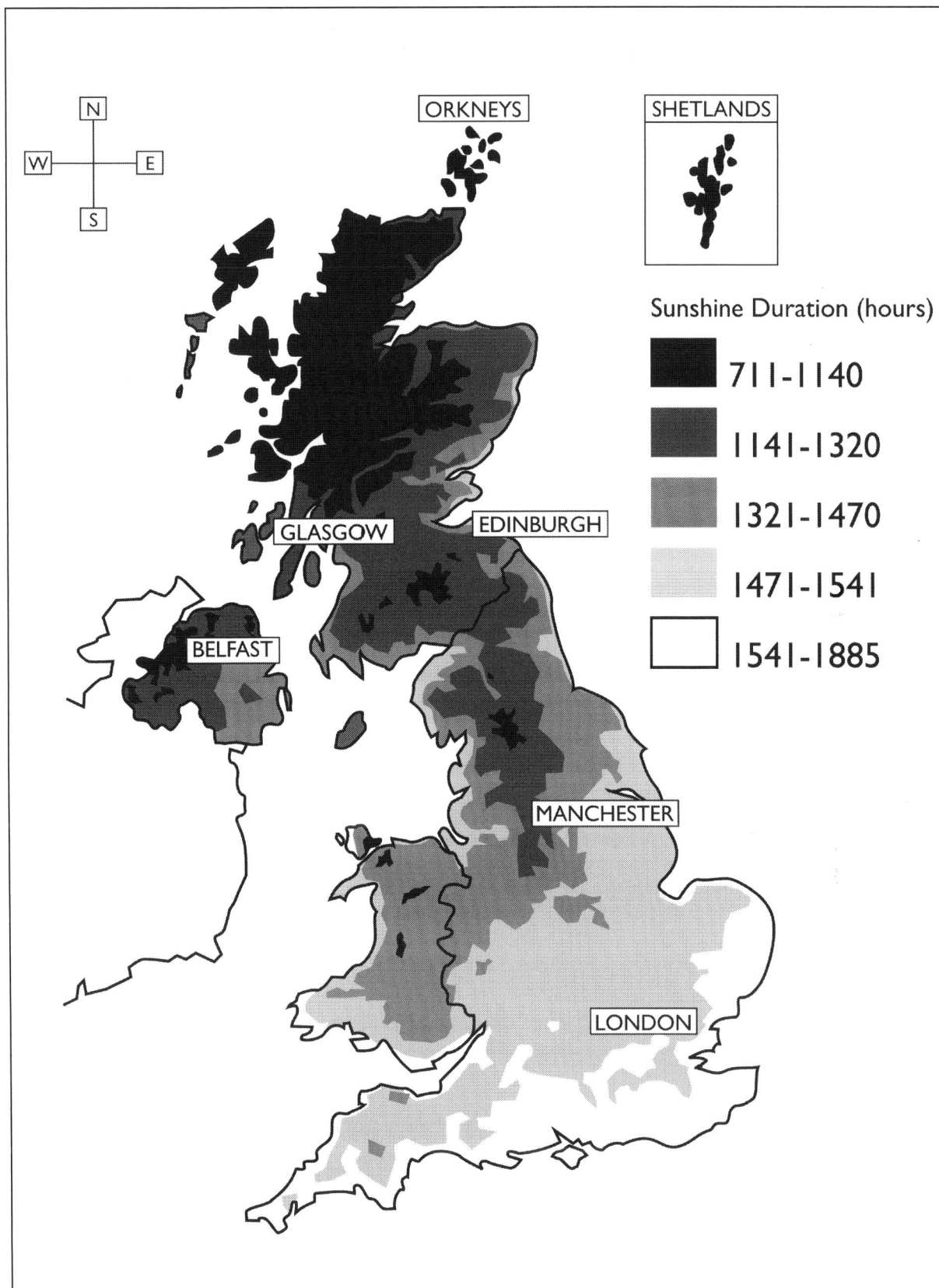

Figure 4. Scotland gets less sun than England because it is so much further north and because it is more exposed to humid westerly and north westerly airstreams which bring cloudy weather and rain. England, on the other hand, is relatively sheltered from the west by Ireland and by the Cumbrian mountains. The sunniest places are on south facing coasts and flat coastal plains. Some sites along the south coast of England from the Isle of Wight eastwards and the Channel Islands record more than 40% of the maximum amount of sunshine possible in a year (1,800 hours out of 4,000). The Shetland Islands only achieve about 24% of the maximum possible sunshine. Map redrawn from Meteorological Office data.

season starts some three weeks earlier and finishes some three weeks later in Scotland compared with southern England while lower air temperatures throughout the summer mean that arms and shoulders are generally much less often exposed. The result is that most people in Scotland get much less exposure to active UVB than in more southern latitudes and so make less vitamin D.

So it is hardly surprising that Scots are twice as likely as southern English to have a low vitamin D level (below either 25 or 40 nmol/L) [5]. The optimum level of vitamin D is now generally accepted to be above 75 nmol/L and in summer 75 per cent of Scots fail to reach this level compared with 57 per cent of people in southern England. While in winter, 92 per cent of Scots fail to reach the optimal level compared to 86 per cent of people in southern England [24]. These figures show that vitamin D insufficiency is a very serious problem in all parts of Britain but Scotland is at the extreme end and so the overall effects of vitamin D insufficiency are very grave indeed for Scotland.

And the problem is likely to get worse and not better unless active steps are taken. People today spend less time outdoors than they used to do and so obtain less vitamin D from the sun than in the past. Television, computers, cars, central heating and air conditioning all encourage indoor living. Wearing of long trousers instead of shorts or skirts by children reduces sun exposure very significantly. Furthermore many cosmetics now contain sunblock that reduces the amount of vitamin D to be obtained by casual exposure to the sun.

Heavy promotion by government of advice to avoid exposure to the sun in the middle of the day, aimed at reducing the risk of skin cancer, has further reduced vitamin D levels. All these factors have combined so that the problem of insufficient vitamin D is more acute now than it has ever been since the first half of the 20th century when heavy air pollution from coal fires and factories prevented UVB rays reaching people in cities and towns. Rickets was then common in European cities, particularly Glasgow and other Scots industrial areas. The steady increase in incidence in the UK of diseases such as multiple sclerosis and diabetes type 1, where vitamin D appears to play a crucial role, may be explained at least in part by these changes in everyday exposure to the sun.

2. Eskimos, Lapps – and Scots

In winter the sun is not strong enough in Scotland, or indeed in any country north of 37° latitude, to make a useful amount of vitamin D. Vitamin D has a half life *in vivo* of two to three months [25] and so winter levels of vitamin D are unlikely to remain optimal for people in Scotland except perhaps for a few individuals who build up large stores of the vitamin by regular sunbathing in summer, or go for a winter sunshine holiday.

Eskimos (Inuit), who live above the Arctic Circle where summers are very short, get most of their vitamin D from their marine diet. Not only fish, but also whale, seal and other marine meats and blubber are a good source of vitamin D. Eskimos, who live inland in Alaska and northern Canada and survive by hunting caribou, trade with others on the coast to obtain concentrated fish oil which is a delicacy for them and makes an important contribution to their diet [26]. Lapps, who also live close to the Arctic Circle, obtain much vitamin D from reindeer meat and stomach contents that is rich in the vitamin because the reindeer themselves eat "moss" (actually a lichen) rich in vitamin D.

In Scotland the "vitamin D winter", the darker months when there is insufficient active UVB for synthesis of the vitamin, lasts four to six weeks longer than in southern England. So stores of vitamin D in the body are more likely to run down to dangerously low levels during the winter in Scotland than in England, as has been well documented [5].

Changes in diet in Scotland over the last 100 years have probably made the winter shortage of vitamin D today more extreme than before, at least in coastal areas of the country. In 1868 Hutchison recorded the diets of agricultural labourers in Scotland and at that time fish appear to have played a larger part than meat in the diet of the families of a ploughman and a shepherd, two of the examples given [27]. We cannot generalise from two observations but for many Scots, especially those living in coastal areas, fish used to be a more important part of the diet than it is now. Salted and smoked herring (kippers), which are rich in vitamin D, were a more common part of the Scots diet in the past. Now herring stocks are seriously depleted and some local races of herring have been completely wiped out while white fish stocks have also been seriously reduced [28].

This has happened since the use of steam trawlers began in the second half of the 19th century. Use of steam engines allowed boats to go further, survive more hostile weather and tow bigger nets. New markets for Scots' fish opened up in England following development of the railways and fish stocks were devastated [28]. Now fish is no longer the cheap food that once nourished the poor and provided an important quantity of vitamin D. (See Chapter 6 for more about changes in fish stocks and its possible effects on diseases in the north Atlantic islands). In Scandinavia fish has remained a more important part of the diet and many more people regularly take a supplement of cod liver oil (which is rich in vitamin D) as a "health tonic".

Nowadays most healthy people in the UK get only about 5% of the vitamin D they need from their diet – fish, meat, margarine and eggs being the main sources. Those who regularly eat oily fish may get a little more, but at most they can get only 10% of the vitamin D they need for optimum health this way. In any case current official advice from the UK Food Standards Agency is to eat fish no more than three times per week because sea water is polluted with toxins such as lead that are taken up by fish.

Fish is also the best source of omega-3 fatty acids which have a number of health benefits. So fish meals three times a week are highly recommended. A fish oil supplement such as cod liver oil or halibut liver oil can also be highly recommended as a source of both omega-3 fatty acids and vitamin D. However the recommended dose of these fish oils does not provide enough vitamin D to enable optimum levels to be reached. Purified omega-3 fish oils, which are widely promoted, generally contain no vitamin D. So fish oils of all kinds need to be supplemented with vitamin D in another form. Although food generally provides little vitamin D it is nevertheless an important source of vitamin D for people who get little exposure to the sun and may prevent the most extreme ill health caused by insufficient D, such as rickets or osteomalacia. Vegetarians, especially vegans, are at particularly high risk of the more severe types of D insufficiency and it is specially important for them to actively seek exposure to the sun and/or take a vitamin D supplement. An optimal level of vitamin D can only be obtained in Scotland by taking a supplement.

3. Remarkable list of D diseases

Diseases associated with insufficient vitamin D, and now believed to be caused at least in part by D-insufficiency, include: multiple sclerosis, diabetes (1 and 2), hypertension, arthritis, tuberculosis, several different types of cancer, cardiovascular disease, pre-eclampsia (a serious complication of pregnancy), dental decay and gum disease, Crohn's disease and other autoimmune diseases, as well as the classic bone diseases, rickets, osteoporosis and osteomalacia [20, 29-31].

Until recently it was hard to believe that vitamin D could have an important role in so many different diseases. Researchers found it difficult to understand how one factor, insufficient vitamin D, could even be a partial cause of so many different diseases. However we now know that vitamin D is processed locally in more than 30 different tissues and organs of the human body. It has been shown to act on tissues causing activation of 1000 different genes, differentiation of cells, and regulated cell death (apoptosis) [32].

Insufficient vitamin D might cause disease in a particular organ and not another as a result of timing, genetic background and other circumstances. Detailed biological evidence explains the mechanism of action of vitamin D in heart disease [33, 34], cancer [35, 36] and a number of other diseases not just those of bone.

4. The 'Scottish effect' – an explanation

Deaths from all causes among people of working age are more frequent in Scotland than any other Western European country – see Figure 5. Furthermore Scotland has a higher overall mortality than England and Wales that cannot be explained by differences in smoking, alcohol consumption, poverty or other established risk factors. This hitherto unexplained excess mortality in Scotland compared with England and other industrial countries has been called the "Scottish effect" [1, 2, 13].

The health deficit in Scotland effects people in all walks of life. In the 1980s, for example, Scots from all social classes died earlier than people in the same social class as them in the rest of the UK. The Scottish Council Foundation's report on The Possible Scot [2] puts it this way: "The relative position of Scotland as a whole has worsened at a time when average measures of income, unemployment and housing standards have improved. Scotland's health is worse across the board than in equivalent areas of the United Kingdom. That suggests there may be factors other than relative deprivation that underlie Scotland's poor figures. There may be an additional Scottish Effect. The existence and nature of this effect urgently requires further exploration..."

Different levels of vitamin D in the Scottish and English populations, caused ultimately by differences between the Scottish and English climate, could explain the Scottish effect [5]. This explanation does not appear to have been considered before because low vitamin D levels have only recently been recognised as an important risk factor for cancer, heart disease, hypertension and other common ills. Several recent reports on health in Scotland make little or no mention of vitamin D showing that the seriousness of vitamin D deprivation in Scotland and its consequences are poorly understood by UK health professionals including high profile nutritionists and food experts [2, 12, 14-17].

Being born in Scotland and spending early years in the country appears to be enough to increase the risk of

Figure 5. Life expectancy at birth (1995-1997) by country and British Government region. Notice regions are in a rough north/south gradient, but care must be taken not to over-interpret this because the figures have not been corrected for smoking, alcohol or poverty. Nevertheless Scotland has the lowest life expectancy of all UK countries or regions. Source ONS

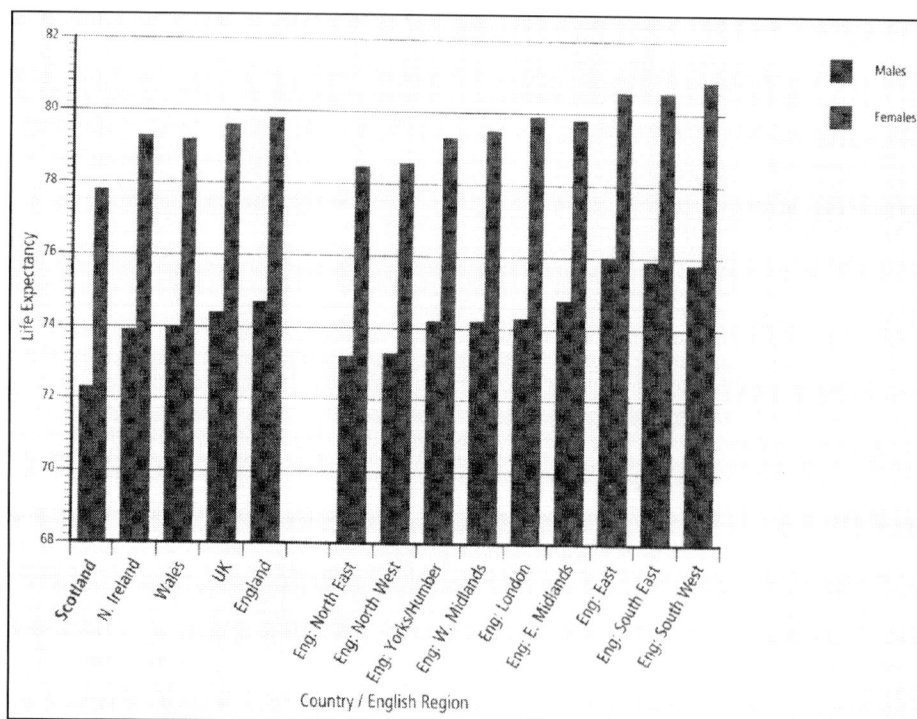

premature death. People born in Scotland but moving to England have a greater risk of death (higher standardised mortality rate or SMR) than people born and living in England [37]. While people born in England but moving to Scotland have a lower risk of death (lower SMR) than native Scots, born and bred [38]. This suggests that there is some factor in the early life of many Scots that leads to a premature death. Insufficient vitamin D during pregnancy, growth and development could be the missing factor and evidence reviewed below supports such an explanation.

5. An early death in Scotland: Mortality studies

During the decade 1988-98 life expectancy in Scotland was consistently lower than other EC countries – the only exception was Portuguese men whose life expectancy is marginally lower than Scottish men [1]. Scotland had higher premature mortality rates than all other countries in Europe between 1991 and 1997 and a higher premature mortality rate than every region in the UK including regions in the north of England [39]. Even so health has actually been improving in Scotland, but not as rapidly as in other European countries, and at the present rate Scotland will never catch up.

Premature mortality in the Strathclyde (Glasgow) region, where deprivation is greatest, is particularly high. However high deprivation in this area cannot by itself account for the difference between Scotland and England because all Scottish regions except Grampian had above average premature mortality for the UK (1991-97). Indeed the difference in life expectancy between Scotland and England is increasing. In 1981 life expectancy was 12% lower in Scotland than in England increasing to 15% lower in 2001 [1].

In the past the higher premature mortality in Scotland has been explained by a higher level of deprivation in Scotland [40]. However, after adjustments are made for differences in deprivation, age and sex structure of the population premature mortality in Scotland was still 8.2% greater than England in 2001 [1]. And when the most deprived areas of Scotland were compared with equally deprived areas of England and Wales premature mortality was found to be 17% higher in Scotland.

Industrial decline has often been given as the reason for Scotland's poor health record. A new report, *The Aftershock of De-industrialisation*, compares the West of Scotland with 20 other old industrial regions in the UK and Europe such as the Ruhr, Alsace-Lorraine and Silesia in Poland as well as Northern Ireland, Tyne and Wear and the Tees Valley [41]. The report finds that mortality in Scotland is comparatively high and the rate of improvement in mortality is relatively slow compared with these other industrial areas, even though Scotland compares favourably when it comes to wealth, unemployment and educational attainment.

The authors consider a number of possible explanations: in particular higher levels of alcohol consumption, smoking among women, obesity, deprivation and possibly greater levels of inequality. The report comes to

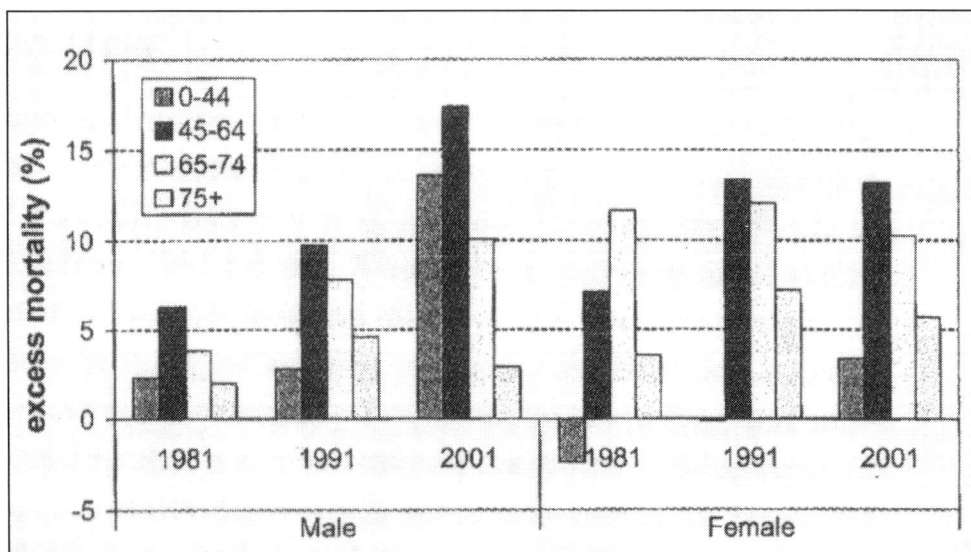

Figure 6. Excess mortality in Scotland compared with England by comparison of mortality rates standardised for deprivation. From *Hanlon* et al., *Journal of Public Health. 27 (2) pp 199-204.*

the overall conclusion that reasons for poor health in the West of Scotland are unclear.

However, there is one factor that the *Aftershock* report does not consider. The West of Scotland is the most northerly of the 20 industrial areas compared in the report. Industrialisation involves moving from rural occupations in the country into cities where work is indoors and workers often live in apartments where they get less exposure to the sun. This factor must have a greater effect in areas that are further north, have a cloudy maritime climate and have a colder air temperature in summer like the west of Scotland.

It might be thought instructive to make a direct comparison of Clydeside with Tyne, Wear and Tees, as can be done with data in the *Aftershock* report. The comparison seems to be appropriate because both are regions where shipbuilding and coal have been dominating industries, and they are so near in distance and latitude it might be thought that there is little difference in sunlight. However there is a large difference in UVB (effective for vitamin D synthesis) received on the west and east of the country, according to measurements made by the National Radiological Protection Board. People in Durham get some 50% more effective UVB than people in Glasgow [23]. This must be because Durham is sheltered by mountains to the north and west which precipitate much of the moisture coming from westerly and north-westerly Atlantic winds, while Glasgow is fully exposed to the wet westerlies.

Other factors such as availability of outdoor play areas for children, sports fields for adults, balconies on blocks of flats, advice about sun exposure, availability of vitamin D supplements for children and adults may all differ critically between the industrial areas being considered in various parts of Europe, and could account for differences in health between them. This suggestion is easily tested by measuring vitamin D levels in people living in these areas. However it will be necessary to study large numbers to obtain a significant result because it is those people at the far end of the statistical distribution who are most deficient in vitamin D and are most likely to show disease.

Looking for the cause of the difference in mortality between Scotland and England we find that Scotland generally has a higher incidence of chronic diseases that are caused at least in part by insufficient vitamin D. Indeed insufficient vitamin D and the northern location that causes it may explain most of the otherwise unaccounted differences in health between the two UK regions, and also may account for some of the difference between Scottish industrial areas and those on the continent. In the sections that follow I examine how the incidence or prevalence of several major diseases varies between Scotland and England together with evidence that suggests the differences may be caused at least in part by vitamin D insufficiency.

Chapter 2:
Scotland's major killers

1. Heart and blood vessel disease

People who live in Scotland have a greater risk of heart and blood vessel disease and consequent death compared with people almost anywhere else in Europe. Only the Finns suffer from more cardiovascular disease than the Scots. Insufficient vitamin D is now known to be a risk factor for heart disease, hypertension and stroke and these diseases account for a substantial part of the "Scottish effect" – the difference in mortality between Scotland and England.

Finnish men currently have the European record for heart disease previously held by Scottish men, while Scottish women have retained the highest mortality rate for heart disease in Europe since the 1950s [42]. And apart from Portugal, Scotland has the highest mortality rate from stroke in Western Europe [42].

The high incidence of stroke in Portugal may be due, at least in part, to their high consumption of salt, especially salt fish. Salt is well known as a risk factor for raised blood pressure and stroke. In view of the multi-factorial cause of most chronic diseases, and particularly cardiovascular and cerebrovascular disease (stroke), it is perhaps surprising that correlations with vitamin D levels, north/south location, latitude, and hours of sunlight, all stand out as clearly as they do.

The high rate of heart disease in Scotland cannot be explained by conventional risk factors [43]. Richard Mitchell and colleagues warn [43]: "Greater prevalence of individual IHD [ischaemic heart disease] risk factors among the Scots explains relatively little of their higher rates of heart disease, relative to the English. This means that current policy interventions aimed at behavioural change are unlikely to narrow the IHD gap between these neighbouring nations." It seems likely that the poor heart health of Scots is caused by some other risk factor that has not been considered up to now.

In 1995 an Australian, Robert Scragg, brought together significant observations suggesting that vitamin D may be an important risk factor for heart disease [44]. He argued cogently that studies of latitude, altitude, and season consistently suggest that sunlight is a significant risk factor in heart disease [45-48]. Scragg noted differences in heart disease and hypertension between Scotland and England which could not be accounted for by recognised risk factors [49].

North/south gradient in heart disease

The "north/south gradient" in heart disease and stroke continued to be a puzzle and could not be accounted for entirely by known variables leaving climate as a possible explanation of the remaining residual variance [50, 51]. Morris and colleagues have made many investigations of risk factors for heart disease. However the relationship with climate was obscured for them because one of the variables they used for explanatory purposes was hypertension (raised blood pressure) which itself has been shown to display a north/south gradient [52, 53].

Raised blood pressure has been known for some time to be associated with lower levels of sun exposure and/or insufficient vitamin D in the diet, and this relationship has been confirmed by a recent study showing that plasma levels of vitamin D* are inversely associated with the risk of high blood pressure [53]. Furthermore blood pressure (systolic) in normal healthy people has also been found to vary with their vitamin D level – people with higher blood pressure have lower vitamin D [54].

So the overall north/south difference in heart disease plus hypertension that may be attributed to an unknown geographical factor, probably sunlight, must be substantially larger than the residual originally considered by Morris. This suggests an important role for sunlight in cardiovascular disease that has not hitherto been widely recognised. Confirmation that a biochemical difference lies behind the north/south gradient of heart disease in Europe comes from a recent study of low-density lipoprotein (LDL) that, with the exception of Italy, shows a similar gradient across the continent. LDL is an established risk factor for atherosclerosis and hence for coronary artery and cerebrovascular disease [55].

Men born in the northern part of the UK who move to the south have lower risks of cardiovascular disease and death compared with those who remain at home in the north. Those migrating south acquire similar risks to those born and living in the south, while men born in the south who move north increase their risk of cardiovascular disease and death [56]. Similarly men living in Scotland have been found to have a higher mean blood pressure than

---

* all measurements of vitamin D referred to in the book are made as 25(OH)D which is now well established as the standard.

men living in the south of England [49], while the place where the men spent most of their adult lives had a much stronger influence on their blood pressure than the place where they were born and brought up.

South Asians living in Scotland but born elsewhere might be reassured because they do not show an excess mortality from heart disease compared with native Scots. However this is only because the inhospitable nature of the Scots environment affects them equally as it does native Scots. South Asians living in Scotland have a substantial excess of heart disease compared with South Asians living in England, so mirroring the excess heart disease in Scots compared with the English [38].

Similar regional variation has been found for other cardiovascular and respiratory risk factors in the UK [57]. These results are what would be expected if sun exposure were a major factor in heart disease and hypertension in Scotland. Indeed almost half of the variance in mortality from heart disease in different districts of the UK can be explained by variation in hours of sunshine suggesting directly that greater exposure to the sun might save lives [58].

Observations from the NHANES study (National Health and Nutrition Examination Survey) provide support for a general effect of vitamin D in maintaining blood vessels in a good operational state [59]. NHANES investigators found that low serum vitamin D levels are associated with a higher prevalence of peripheral arterial disease. By way of explanation of this effect they remarked: "Vitamin D is an inhibitor of the renin-angiotensin system and has anti-inflammatory and anticoagulant properties."

The interpretation offered here that vitamin D insufficiency plays a substantial role in regional variation in the incidence of heart disease and accounts for the north/south gradient in the UK might be tested by re-examination of stored blood and data held by the British Regional Heart Study. I first suggested this to leaders of BRHS in 2004 but funds were not then available to test it, perhaps because the importance of vitamin D was not so widely appreciated at that time. It seems likely that regional variation in vitamin D levels may be an important missing factor in their account of heart disease in Britain.

2. Blood pressure and stroke – the quiet killers

The lower average levels of vitamin D in Scotland compared with England can account at least in part for the very high incidence of stroke north of the border. Low levels of vitamin D are now recognised to be an important risk factor for raised blood pressure, which is a major cause of stroke. Raised blood pressure (hypertension) is also recognised as a major risk factor for heart disease earning it the title of the quiet killer.

The risk factors generally recognised for raised blood pressure are the same as for heart disease and stroke: smoking, diabetes, diet (insufficient fruit and vegetables), lack of exercise, obesity and age. To these we must now add low levels of vitamin D. The effect of insufficient vitamin D on blood pressure may explain the north/south gradient for both stroke and heart disease in the UK [51].

The involvement of sunlight and vitamin D in determining blood pressure was elaborated by Stephen Rostand in 1997 [52]. He showed that differences in sun exposure and vitamin D levels could explain seasonal changes in blood pressure, variation of blood pressure with latitude, and differences in blood pressure between races. His astute analysis has recently been supported by two major epidemiological studies. Some 1,800 individuals were followed for four years in the Health Professionals Follow-up study and the Nurses Health Study [53]. Men with low levels of vitamin D (less than 15 ng/ml or 37.5 nmol/L) were six times more likely to have raised blood pressure than those with high levels of vitamin D (greater than 30 ng/ml or 75 nmol/L). While women with low D were 2.67 times more likely than women with high D to have raised blood pressure.

This finding was confirmed by another two studies. The third National Health and Nutrition Examination Survey found that people with a vitamin D level greater than 32 ng/ml or 80 nmol/L had a blood pressure 20% less than people who had vitamin D levels less than 20 ng/ml or 50 nmol/L [54]. Differences between this study and the Health Professionals and Nurses study may be accounted for by the way the blood samples were taken, since there is a large seasonal variation in blood levels of vitamin D that can influence findings when it is not fully controlled. Another study of people over 65 in Amsterdam found that those with raised parathyroid hormone (which is generally elevated when vitamin D levels are reduced) also tended to have raised blood pressure [60].

Additional evidence showing that blood pressure is strongly influenced by vitamin D levels comes from clinical trials showing that blood pressure may be lowered by exposing the body repeatedly to UV or by taking a vitamin D supplement. Whole body radiation with UVB on a sunbed three times a week for several weeks has been reported to reduce both systolic and diastolic blood pressure by an average 6 mms of mercury [61] Controls exposed to UVA radiation, which does not induce production of vitamin D, showed no reduction in blood pressure.

A vitamin D supplement of 800 IUs per day plus calcium for eight weeks, lowered systolic blood pressure by 5 mm of mercury in 81% of people taking it, whereas calcium alone reduced blood pressure in only 47% of people treated [62]. Other trials of alphacalcidol, a synthetic form of calcitriol, the active hormone form of vitamin D, have shown that this too may reduce blood pressure of men aged 61 to 65 by an average of 9 mmm mercury [63].

Increased blood pressure is closely associated with an increase in risk of stroke [64]. Furthermore lowering blood pressure is well known to reduce the risk of a first or subsequent stroke [65, 66]. Since vitamin D lowers blood pressure it may be expected that vitamin D might also be effective in preventing stroke. Indeed people over 65 in Finland with a low intake of vitamin D or a low serum level of the vitamin have been found to be at increased risk of stroke when observed over a 10 year period [67]; and a study in Cambridge found that 44 patients who had an acute stroke had reduced levels of vitamin D compared with controls [68]. A population based study in Japan has found that the highest incidence of stroke occurs in the spring when vitamin D levels are at their lowest regardless of age, sex and other risk factors and similar seasonal occurrence of stroke has been found in many other countries [69].

So it seems very likely that the high incidence of stroke in Scotland could be reduced if levels of vitamin D in the population could be raised. Vitamin D may also be effective in lowering blood pressure and improving function of blood vessels in stroke patients. Dr Miles Witham and others are currently testing this in a trial at Dundee University.

3. Heart failure – vitamin D can help

Heart failure is a major cause of illness and death in Scotland, as it is in most industrial countries. In 2003 there were estimated to be 40,000 men and 45,000 women aged 45 or over with heart failure in Scotland. This number is forecast to be increasing rapidly with an extra 20,000 people in Scotland developing heart failure by 2020, if age changes in the Scottish population occur as expected. Hospital admissions for heart failure in Scotland are forecast to increase by 52% for men and 16 for women by 2020 [70].

Heart failure appears to be more common in Glasgow than in the English West Midlands suggesting that it might account in part for the "Scottish effect" on mortality. Dr Theresa McDonagh of the Western Infirmary, Glasgow, found that 2.9% of a sample of 1,640 people aged 25 to 74 from north Glasgow had definite heart failure, measured as left ventricular systolic dysfunction [71]. This compares with 1.8% of 3960 people aged 45 plus years from the West Midlands with definite heart failure studied by doctors at Birmingham University [72].*

The importance of vitamin D as a risk factor in heart disease is not yet widely appreciated although it is now well established in clinical studies [73]. Zittermann, for example, has reviewed the evidence [74] and Michos and Blumenthal have commented in some detail in an editorial in the journal *Circulation* [75].

Vitamin D appears to be effective as an anti-inflammatory in heart failure. Zittermann [33, 76-80], Weber [81], Vieth [82], and Schleitoff [80] provide detailed explanations of how they believe vitamin D insufficiency acts as a risk factor for cardiovascular events and for heart failure. Mechanisms by which vitamin D may act to prevent heart disease include: inhibition of vascular smooth muscle proliferation, inhibition of vascular calcification, down regulation of pro-inflammatory cytokines, the up regulation of anti-inflammatory cytokines, and action as a negative regulator of the renin-angiotensin system. And recently vitamin D has been shown to directly modulate vascular tone by reducing calcium influx into endothelial cells, so reducing production of endothelium-derived contraction factors [83].

Vitamin D may also protect against atherosclerosis, the basic process that causes blocking of arteries. Low levels of vitamin D in blood are associated with a higher prevalence of peripheral artery disease in the US National Health and Nutrition Examination Survey (NHANES) [59]. Furthermore a randomised trial undertaken in Dundee has found that a single large dose of 100,000 IUs vitamin D2 improves endothelial function in patients with diabetes type 2 [84].

An impaired vitamin D and parathyroid hormone axis seems to be a part of the heart failure syndrome [81] and treatment with vitamin D as an anti-inflammatory appears to be effective in patients with heart failure [80]. Patients may enter a vicious circle of low vitamin D levels and high inflammatory cytokines if vitamin D deficiency persists. However, as Vieth points out, it is ambitious to hope for a dramatic beneficial effect of vitamin D at a late stage in

---

* The Scottish doctors used a stricter criterion for the left ventricular ejection fraction of <30% compared with <40% used by the English doctors. Furthermore the Scottish sample included people under 45 years of age. It seems that a true like-for-like comparison of the results of the two surveys would produce an even greater difference between Glasgow and the West Midlands. However people in north Glasgow cannot be taken as representative of Scotland as a whole, nor West Midlanders of England as a whole. Also there could have been other technical differences between the methods used by the two groups. So these findings, while giving a possible indication, cannot be safely generalised to Scotland or England as a whole.

heart failure [82]. Greater benefits may occur if vitamin D is used in an early stage of heart disease or for prevention.

4. Heart failure in infants: tip of an iceberg

Children with no obvious structural defect of the heart may suffer from heart failure caused by vitamin D deficiency, which would be fatal without modern treatments. This type of heart muscle failure appears to be more common in Scotland than in other parts of the British Isles. The case frequency in Scotland is 1.27 per 100,000 compared with 0.71 in southern England [85]. However the numbers in this survey are relatively small (12 cases in Scotland and 36 in southern England) so the difference between the two countries could be a matter of chance.

Heart failure, heart muscle disease, and myocarditis in children could all be caused by vitamin D deficiency says Dr David Sane in correspondence in the journal *Circulation* [86]. He points to evidence consistent with the idea that insufficient exposure to the sun may be a risk factor for heart failure in children. A higher incidence of unexplained heart failure (that is heart failure induced by heart muscle disease without any anatomical defect) is found in children in New England compared with the central south western United States [87]. Also black children in the US, who are more prone to vitamin D deficiency, have higher rates of cardiomyopathy than whites [87].

Dr Sane suggests that paediatric patients with heart failure should be screened for vitamin D deficiency. Replying to Dr Sane's letter in *Circulation*, Dr Michael Burch and colleagues suggest that "as many as 25% of cases of infant heart failure in South East England may be caused by vitamin D deficiency and conceivably it may be the most common cause of infant heart failure in breast fed, dark skinned infants" [88]. In the UK one third of these children have been found to die or require heart transplantation within a year of presentation [85]. Heart failure may also account for a proportion of unexplained sudden deaths of infants, that is cot deaths, also known as sudden infant death syndrome (SIDS).

A study of 16 cases of infant heart failure from hospitals in south east England has brought wider recognition for the disease which, apart from a few isolated cases, seems to have been overlooked until now [89]. The 16 cases studied by Dr Burch and colleagues at Great Ormond Street Hospital for Children and other London Hospitals all came from families of Asian or African ethnic origin and all the infants were breast-fed. Most presented at the end of winter (February to May) when vitamin D levels are lowest. Breast milk contains very little vitamin D, except when the mother is very well supplemented with the vitamin, whereas formula milk is fortified with vitamin D.

Dr Michael Burch, the paediatric cardiologist who drew the 16 cases of infant heart failure together, said: "Life threatening heart failure occurring in babies in 21st century London, just from failure to be given a vitamin, is a shocking fact."

The infants had all been admitted as emergencies to intensive care units – 10 were suffering from heart failure and six had suffered a cardiac arrest. All the infants were profoundly deficient in calcium and vitamin D and had high levels of parathyroid hormone. Ten of the infants had radiological evidence of rickets. Three died and two were scheduled for heart transplants. However all the survivors, including those scheduled for transplant, responded to vitamin D and calcium plus anti-heart-failure medication, and made slow but good recoveries without transplantation.

Finding 16 cases over six years in the south east of England alone suggests that there are likely to be many more in the UK. The London doctors point out that the underlying problem is probably even more extensive: "It deserves emphasis that the infants in this series had overt and severe clinical heart failure, and it seems very likely that many infants from these ethnic groups would have had undetected sub-clinical, but potentially important, cardiac abnormality during the same era... It is concerning that none of the mothers or infants were receiving the recommended vitamin D supplementation".

So vitamin D deficiency is an important, and possibly even common, cause of illness in infants in the UK. One in five Asian schoolchildren examined in Glasgow were found to suffer from low calcium in their blood or X-ray evidence of rickets compared with only one in ten in England [90]. Vitamin D deficiency has not until now been well recognised as a cause of infant heart failure. Large studies have been made of cardiomyopathy (heart muscle disease) in infants from North America and Australia but vitamin D deficiency does not seem to have been considered as a possible cause of infant heart failure in these cases [91, 92].

Mothers and infants in Scotland, as in England, have not generally been given a vitamin D supplement in recent years. The lack of supplements for mothers and infants is a result of failings in government policy which can only be described as negligent [93]. More details are given below, see: *Westminster bungles supply of infant vitamin, and, Rickets and fractures: Asians in Glasgow.*

Summary: Vitamin D insufficiency plays an important part in raised blood pressure, and in heart failure of both infants and old people. A higher incidence of vitamin D insufficiency in Scotland compared with England could explain the higher incidence of heart disease and stroke in Scotland and account in part for the " Scottish effect". An increase in vitamin D from sunlight and from supplements or food in Scotland might reasonably be expected to lower mortality from heart disease and stroke.

5. Cancer: increased risk

International studies suggest that people living at high latitudes, such as northern Europe, are at increased risk of death from many cancers including the most common types: breast, colon, pancreatic, prostate, and ovarian cancers, and Hodgkin's lymphoma [30, 94]. Scotland follows this pattern and has a relatively high incidence of cancer compared with most other European countries – see Figure 7 [42]. Countries at high latitudes, such as Scotland, have a relatively low intensity of sunlight and a relatively short summer season and so the inhabitants obtain less exposure to UVB, and less vitamin D, which we now know makes them more vulnerable to cancer.

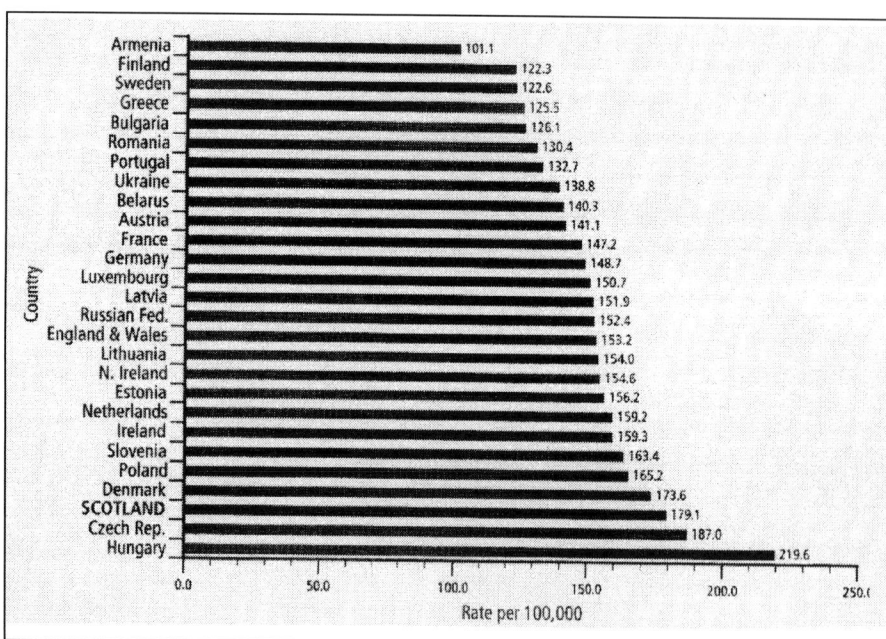

Figure 7. Mortality rates (age-standardised) for all malignancies per 100,000 population for selected European countries. The large numbers of smokers in Scotland ensures that Scotland comes low in this list but that is only part of the story. Source WHO

Overall the cancer incidence in Scottish men is 16% above that of English men and cancer incidence in Scottish women 13% above that of English women [95]. Much of this difference may be accounted for by differences in smoking, alcohol consumption and possibly obesity [42] which vary geographically in complicated ways. However mortality of Scottish smokers in Renfrew and Paisley from lung cancer is greater per cigarette smoked than it is for English or American smokers [96]. This hint that there may be a geographical factor, such as ultra-violet radiation, that acts as an additional risk factor for smoking is supported by a study showing that the geographical relationship persists in a study of smoking in 111 countries [97].

Individual exposure to the sun and uptake of vitamin D can vary almost as much from personal habits as from latitude even in a sub-tropical climate [98]. The interaction of several risk factors leads to considerable regional variation in cancer incidence within Scotland and England tending to mask any north/south effect on incidence that may generally be found elsewhere over larger ranges of latitude. Even so some cancers have been found to be especially frequent in Scotland.

The mortality for breast cancer in Scotland is close to the European maximum [42]. Other observations support the suggestion that the reason for this is low levels of vitamin D. Women who do not get regular exposure to sunlight, and do not get much vitamin D from other sources, have a significantly higher incidence of breast cancer [94, 99, 100]. Women in the lowest quartile for serum vitamin D have been found to have a risk of breast cancer five times higher than those in the highest quartile for serum vitamin D.

Vitamin D programmes genes and cell death

Scottish rates for bowel (colorectal) cancer were the highest in Europe until the 1970s and remain high, although Ireland, Denmark and Austria now have similar high mortality rates for bowel cancer. The incidence of bowel cancer in Europe varies about four fold when the highest and lowest incidence rates are compared and internationally rates vary 60-fold [101]. A UK survey of people aged 50-69 years found that bowel cancer is almost twice as common in the Scottish areas surveyed (Grampian, Tayside and Fife) compared with the English areas (Coventry and Warwickshire) [102]. Many studies using different methodologies have now established a link between sun exposure, vitamin D in the diet or serum, and bowel cancer [94, 100, 103].

The suggestion that one substance, vitamin D, could have such a profound effect on cancers of several types was at first greeted with disbelief by some scientists. But we should no longer be surprised. Receptors for vitamin D have been found in almost every tissue in the body. Vitamin D is processed locally into its active hormone form in each organ or tissue in a way that is individually specified by the genes.

In its active hormone form 1,25(OH)2D, vitamin D controls more than 1000 genes including genes responsible for the regulation of cellular proliferation, programmed cell death (apoptosis), and growth of blood vessels [32] . This proliferation of blood vessels known as angiogenesis occurs when tumours sequester their own blood supply enabling them to grow even faster. Vitamin D also decreases cellular proliferation of both normal and cancer cells and induces them to differentiate into their final form – rather than remain as intermediate forms which are at risk of developing into cancer cells [35, 104].

There is now a consensus of international experts who agree that the risk of cancer is likely to be reduced by increasing the average individual's exposure to the sun and/or by taking a vitamin D supplement of about 1000 IUs per day or more [9-11, 20, 30, 94, 105-107]. This conclusion is backed up by the results of a double blind randomised trial in women who had an average age of 67 years [11]. The women were given 1100 IUs of vitamin D/day with the original intention of studying benefit in preventing fractures but it was found after four years that there was a 77% reduction in cancer among the women taking vitamin D compared with those taking a placebo.

William Grant, a former NASA scientist now dedicated to work on vitamin D and sunlight, has estimated that 17 different types of cancer are sensitive to UV, that is to say insufficient vitamin D puts a person at increased risk of contracting the cancer and/or dying from it [108]. This number is obtained by comparing figures for mortality from cancer with intensity of UV radiation in different countries, states or regions. The method is controversial but has produced results that are broadly consistent with other methods and so compels our attention. Indeed it may be that insufficient vitamin D is a risk factor for most, if not all, types of cancer because some cancers are too rare to be assessed by Grant's method of analysis. However a more conservative assessment concludes that only in the case of bowel and colon cancer, breast cancer and lymphoma (lymph gland cancer) is there clear evidence that insufficient vitamin D is a risk factor [107, 109].

There have been relatively few negative findings on the relationship between cancer and vitamin D. However four studies now show that the risk of prostate cancer is not reduced in people with higher blood levels of vitamin D [110]. Risk of multiple myeloma may be increased by sun exposure according to one study which also found that risk of the more common lymphoma is reduced by sun exposure [107]. This is the first such finding for multiple myeloma and so should be confirmed before it is accepted while the reduction of risk of lymphoma associated with increased sun exposure has been found in three other studies.

Cancer deaths could be reduced by 14 to 19% in the UK if everyone took a supplement of 1000 IUs of vitamin D per day, according to Dr Grant's calculations [108]. Simply going to live in a sunnier country such as the southern United States may reduce the risk of dying from cancer by 50% or more, according to Dr Grant. For residents of Scotland who do not wish to emigrate to sunnier climes a substantial reduction in risk of death from cancer may be obtained if every opportunity is taken to sunbathe without burning or a vitamin D supplement is taken.

Summary: Scotland has a high incidence of cancer, which may account in part for the "Scottish effect". Northern latitude, low sun exposure and low vitamin D levels are associated with a high risk of cancer. Vitamin D has been shown to reduce cancer risk in at least one trial. Boosting vitamin D levels in Scotland can be expected to reduce the incidence of cancer substantially, reducing mortality in a step-change.

Chapter 3:
Scotland's bane: the epidemic of immune system diseases

1. The silent epidemic

Three autoimmune diseases, multiple sclerosis, diabetes type 1, and Crohn's disease occur more frequently in Scotland than in England. A fourth autoimmune disease, rheumatoid arthritis, has a greater prevalence in the United Kingdom than in other European countries. These four common diseases, the "Big Four", occur as a result of the body's own immune system attacking other body tissues causing progressive and devastating illness. Scientific evidence now suggests that vitamin D and/or sunlight, especially in early life, may protect against the big four and that insufficient vitamin D is the common factor linking these diseases.

Taken together these four diseases can be seen to be part of a silent epidemic of autoimmune disease. Silent because it is not widely understood that the big four diseases are linked and that the epidemic may involve dozens of other autoimmune diseases, some rare. The epidemic of autoimmune disease appears to be a worldwide phenomenon of our industrial age, but Scotland is particularly badly afflicted. Looking at multiple sclerosis alone the figures show that Scotland is worse affected than anywhere else in the world [29, 111-113].

Furthermore autoimmune diseases appear to be increasing in incidence year on year but the seriousness of the threat is not fully realised. The incidence of multiple sclerosis, diabetes type 1 and Crohn's disease are all increasing, while there is insufficient data on rheumatoid arthritis to know whether the incidence is changing or not. Asthma, a related immune system disease, is also increasing steadily.

The reason for the increase seems to be our new ways of living, in particular modern life indoors, out of the sun. These diseases are increasing in children who now get much less exposure to the sun than they used to. Children get less exposure because fashion now dictates long trousers even for young children in both summer and winter. As a result exposure of a child's body to the sun may be reduced by a third or more. Greater use of cars, time spent indoors watching TV and playing computer games all reduce the time spent outdoors. Use of suncreams and advice aimed at preventing skin cancer further reduces exposure to the sun. Excess intake of calories and insufficient exercise may also play a part in the increase in autoimmune disease.

Recognition of a common link in the increase in immune system disease, and of an epidemic that extends beyond the big four, comes from studies of thyroid disease in Scotland. Hunter and colleagues found a twofold increase in autoimmune disease of the thyroid in young people on Tayside during the 1990s. They remark that their findings suggest "an increase in autoimmune thyroid disease, similar to the rising prevalence of type 1 diabetes, possibly indicating a rising prevalence of autoimmunity in young people" [114, 115]. These immune system diseases make a substantial contribution to the Scottish effect, the excess of chronic disease that plagues the country.

Vitamin D modulates the immune system

When self tolerance of body tissues breaks down as it does in autoimmune disease certain cells in the immune system called T helper cells become activated, perhaps as the result of an environmental trigger such as infection or perhaps because the immune system itself has failed to mature normally. The T helper cells then attack normal body tissues causing chronic inflammation and increasing damage as the disease progresses [116-118]. The common mechanism of these four diseases has been pointed out by a number of researchers and details have been well worked out in animal studies [119-122].

T helper cells have receptors for vitamin D that enable the vitamin to interact with these cells and reduce their activity. Vitamin D also "modulates" the immune system in other important ways. It suppresses secretion of melatonin which plays a part in priming T helper cells [123], and promotes secretion of melanocyte stimulating hormone which suppresses T helper cell activity [124]. These mechanisms have been well worked out in genetically modified mice with "model diseases" – that is artificially created diseases that simulate multiple sclerosis, diabetes type 1, rheumatoid arthritis or Crohn's. In all four model diseases vitamin D deficiency has been shown to accelerate disease while supplements of vitamin D suppress the diseases in these experimental animals [122].

At least 80 known autoimmune diseases

One person in 30 suffers from an autoimmune disease of some kind and one new case occurs each year for every 1000 people in the United States [125, 126]. There are more than 80 known autoimmune diseases [127]. Complicated interactions of environment, genes and stage of growth will determine which autoimmune disease a person might develop. The environmental influences are likely to include vitamin D availability at various crucial times in development and growth, diet, and timing of infectious disease.

The most common autoimmune diseases other than the big four and thyroid disease are: vitiligo (a skin disorder causing white patches), glomerulonephritis (a kidney disease), systemic lupus erythematosis (inflammation of connective tissue e.g. skin), biliary cirrhosis (a liver disease), myasthenia gravis (general muscle weakness), and systemic sclerosis (also called scleroderma, affects skin and many other organs) [126]. But there are also a substantial number of relatively rare autoimmune syndromes with exotic names such as Goodpasture's, Addison's, Cogan's, and Sjogren's.

Much of the research on autoimmune diseases focuses on them individually but understanding may be gained by comparing them and considering possible common features. In his classic discussion of how to identify causes of disease from epidemiological observations Bradford Hill suggests that analogy provides a useful means of recognising cause, especially when it is supported by a cogent biological model and experimental evidence [128]. So autoimmune diseases may be considered together as a family of analogous diseases and the question naturally arises whether they may not have a common cause.

Present understanding of multiple sclerosis and diabetes type 1 suggests that insufficient vitamin D or sunlight in early life or later is a cause of these two diseases. So, following the classic reasoning by analogy of Bradford Hill, we can predict that insufficient vitamin D may also be a cause of other autoimmune diseases such as rheumatoid arthritis and inflammatory bowel disease. Likewise the analogy may be extended to the whole family of 80 or more autoimmune diseases. And this leads to the expectation and hope that the same practical measures for prevention may be effective i.e. taking of vitamin D supplements, especially in early life but possibly later too, and greater exposure to the sun.

Indeed this reasoning is already bearing fruit. People with Behçet's syndrome, an allergic condition involving inflammation of the eye together with ulcers in the mouth and on the genitals, have been found to have low levels of vitamin D (25(OH)D) in serum [129]. In one study the serum level of vitamin D in people with Behçet's was found to vary inversely with the amount of toll-like receptors. These receptors are involved in the process of inflammation and are produced in larger amounts by people with Behçet's. When white cells from these people were treated with vitamin D in the test tube the formation of the toll-like receptors was suppressed giving hope that vitamin D might have therapeutic potential for Behçet's disease.

Experimental evidence from mice is now accumulating to support use of vitamin D to prevent and/or treat several autoimmune diseases. Diseases for which there is experimental evidence in animals supporting use of vitamin D for prevention or therapy include systemic lupus erythematosus, allergic encephalomyelitis, collagen induced arthritis, Lyme arthritis, and inflammatory bowel disease [130, 131]. And vitamin D is also beginning to be recognised now as beneficial for treatment of several auto-immune disorders in patients [132].

If the disease model to be considered in relation to Bradford Hill's analogy is the broader category, immune system disease, rather than autoimmune disease, then not only is asthma included but also hay fever, eczema, coeliac disease and other allergies. Vitamin D may well be found to benefit these diseases but, apart from asthma, evidence one way or another is not reviewed in this book.

2. The Big Four

2.1. Multiple sclerosis – a world record for Scotland

Multiple sclerosis is more frequent in Scotland than any other country in the world where its occurrence has been measured. Both the prevalence and incidence of the disease are higher in Scotland than anywhere else [133, 134]. On Tayside (latitude 56.5° north) one person in 300 suffers from MS. As in other locations the disease is more common among women than men: 236 women and 100 men per 100,000 on Tayside are affected by the disease as defined by international criteria (age and sex standardised rates). In the Lothian and Border region [133], in the Grampian region [135] and in Orkney and Shetland [136] prevalence rates are almost as high.

Northern Ireland has a prevalence of MS close to that of Scotland but prevalence in England and Wales is typically half that of Scotland – see figure 8 [134]. Fewer studies have been made of incidence because they are more

Figure 8: Prevalence rates for multiple sclerosis in Scotland are up to twice the rates in England - a comparison of the crude prevalence rates in the most recent studies in Scotland, England and Wales. (From Rothwell and Charlton [133]. Where available the figures quoted are based on the Poser category probable and definite cases. For those studies in which these data are unavailable (marked with *) the figures are based on Allison and Millar criteria, excluding possible cases. References: Shetlands 1974 [137], Orkneys 1983 [136], Aberdeen [135], Lothian 1995 [133], Borders 1995 [133], Rochdale 1988 [138], South east Wales 1988 [139], Cambridge 1990 [140], Sutton 1985 [141], Southampton 1987 [142], Sussex 1991 [143].)

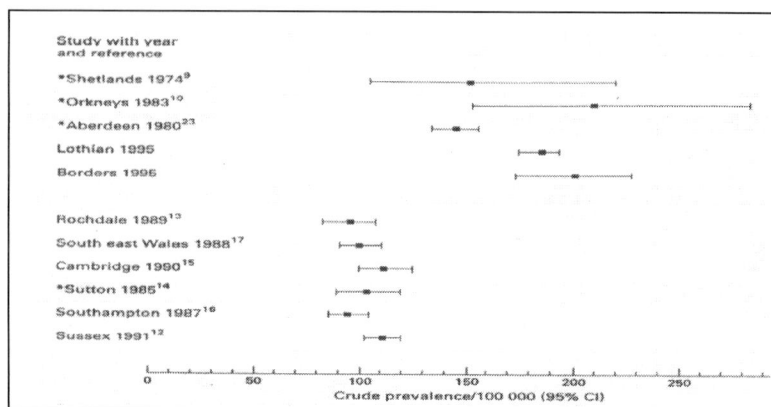

difficult, but in the Lothian and Border areas incidence is between 10 and 12 new cases of MS per 100,000 people per year, the highest incidence rate ever reported anywhere. The higher prevalence of the disease on Tayside suggests that the incidence there could be even higher than in Lothian and Borders but it has not yet been measured.

The high levels of MS in the Celtic fringe (Scotland and Ireland) compared with England have led to suggestions that the disease has a large genetic component. However studies of identical twins with MS have found that in 70-90% of identical pairs only one twin has the disease, suggesting that there is in fact a large environmental component in causation of the disease [133].

Sunshine or moonshine?

The north/south difference in incidence and prevalence of MS in the UK is part of a larger picture showing that MS varies similarly along a latitude gradient in North America, Australia and Europe. This link between climate and MS prevalence was studied in detail in the 1960s by Sir Donald Acheson, the former UK chief medical officer and author of the 1998 Acheson report on inequalities in health [144]. Acheson was able to show that the climatic factor that best explained the distribution of MS was sunshine, especially winter sunshine. He found that the more sunshine there was in a region the less MS there appeared to be.

However Sir Donald's ideas were some 40 years before their time. After presenting his observations at a public meeting in the 1960s, Dr F M R Walshe, the distinguished physician and author of a textbook, *Diseases of the Nervous System,* said to him: "Sunshine? More likely to be moonshine my boy." Sir Donald's evidence was ignored. It was too difficult to comprehend when other parts of the scientific jigsaw were not yet in place. So a generation of scientists pursued more fashionable explanations based on virus infection and genetics.

Measles virus, canine distemper, Epstein-Barr virus and other infections have all been suggested as causes of multiple sclerosis. However intensive investigation over many years has failed to establish the infection hypothesis of MS. Spouses of people with MS are at no greater risk of developing the disease than anyone else, and children in families that adopted a child who developed MS are no more at risk of MS than someone in the general population [133, 145]. This suggests that infectious disease cannot be a necessary and sufficient cause of MS. While it remains possible that infection plays a part in MS it no longer seems likely that it could be a crucial factor without which the disease will not occur [146, 147].

Unifying hypothesis

In November 2004, after a lifetime's work on the disease, Sir Donald Acheson and others proposed a unifying hypothesis at a meeting in London. They suggested that insufficient vitamin D, resulting from inadequate exposure to ultra-violet light, combined with infection are the basic cause of MS. In this proposed scenario infection in a person with a low level of vitamin D triggers an autoimmune reaction attacking the nervous system and initiating MS [144].

However, according to this new theory, infection alone is not sufficient to trigger MS. The immune system must be in disorder as a result of vitamin D insufficiency for the disease to develop. It has also been suggested that vitamin D insufficiency alone may be the cause of MS. Vitamin D may be essential for normal differentiation and adhesion of brain cells known as oligodendrocytes such that when vitamin D is insufficient the brain does not develop normally[148].

Over the last five years or so evidence linking MS with sun exposure has become increasingly compelling. In Australia, where most people in all parts of the country have a similar English/Scots/Irish ancestry, the prevalence of MS (standardised by age) is six fold greater in temperate Tasmania than it is in tropical Queensland and the prevalence of MS is correlated with levels of ultra violet radiation [149]. Further support for the idea that sun exposure in childhood is important for prevention of MS come from studies in Tasmania which have found that two to three hours of exposure to sun per week is associated with a 60% reduction in risk. This association has been confirmed by estimation of lifetime exposure to the sun based on solar damage to skin of the hand [149].

Further evidence suggesting the benefits of sunlight in preventing MS and in ameliorating the disease come from studies of migration. Adult migrants from the UK to a sunny climate such as that of South Africa or Australia reduce their risk of developing MS [144]. Immigrants to the UK from the Indian subcontinent, Africa and the Caribbean rarely develop MS, but their children have a high prevalence of MS comparable to that of the general population of the UK, suggesting that insufficient exposure to the sun in first 20 to 30 years of life increases risk of MS [150]. While British and Irish migrants to Queensland (northern Australia, latitude 120-280 south) which has a sub-tropical climate have a remarkable 75% reduction in their risk of developing MS.

However, the reduction in risk of MS was less for those who migrated to the more southerly and less sunny provinces of Australia reaching zero for those who migrated to Hobart in Tasmania (latitude 420 south) [151, 152]. Those who migrated to Australia before 15 years of age were no less likely to develop MS than those who migrated at a later age leading Dr S R Hammond of the University of Sydney to conclude: "These findings suggest that the risk from environmental factors in multiple sclerosis may operate over a period of many years and not only in childhood and early adult life." [152]

MS less common in outdoor workers

In the UK, MS is less frequent in people who have skin cancer. Since sun exposure is the major factor determining skin cancer this suggests that exposure to the sun in the UK protects against MS [144, 149]. MS is also less common in outdoor workers who obviously obtain greater than average exposure to the sun, suggesting again that risk of the disease may probably be reduced by sun exposure in adult life [153].

Symptoms of multiple sclerosis often have a seasonal pattern which is consistent with the suggestion that vitamin D plays a part in occurrence of the disease. Multiple sclerosis develops intermittently with periods of progressive improvement followed by relapses. Some studies have found that relapses are more likely to occur in spring when levels of vitamin D are lowest [154].

A correlation has also been found between levels of serum vitamin D in the population and the development of lesions in the brains of MS patients detected by imaging [155]. Other more recent work has shown that relapses occur in individual patients when levels of vitamin D are low and parathyroid hormone (which is regulated by the vitamin D level) is high [156]. Furthermore studies on very large numbers of people have shown that those born in late spring or early summer when vitamin D levels are low are at greater risk of developing multiple sclerosis [133].

All these observations taken together provide compelling evidence that multiple sclerosis is caused by insufficient sunlight and/or vitamin D. This is the view that world experts are arriving at having spent long years eliminating other possible explanations. For example, George Ebers, professor of clinical neurology at Oxford University, says that it seems increasingly probable that sunlight or vitamin D is a major environmental risk factor for multiple sclerosis [157]. Regrettably the highly learned SACN committee has not taken this view because they did not have time to make a full review of the evidence, which is essential if an understanding of multiple sclerosis is to be achieved [158].

Trials of vitamin D for MS

Observations of seasonal influences on MS together with the results of migration studies encourage us to hope that increased sun exposure or vitamin D supplements might reduce exacerbations of multiple sclerosis. One large observational study, Nurses Health Study I and II (NHANES), supports this suggestion. Nurses who took a multivitamin supplying an average of about 400 IU vitamin D per day had a 40% reduced risk of developing multiple sclerosis compared with those who had never used a multi-vitamin. Taken in conjunction with everything else we know, the simplest explanation is that the observed benefit was derived from vitamin D. However it is possible that the benefit came from another vitamin in the multi-vitamin mixture [159].

In another trial, magnesium, calcium and cod liver oil supplying 5000 IUs of vitamin D per day were found to reduce the expected number of exacerbations or relapses of MS [160]. Three other very small trials of vitamin D, its derivatives or analogues, have produced equivocal results [161]. A large trial is now needed to collect definitive data and this will need to be financed by government or charitable funds since a drug company could never recoup investment in such a trial.

MS has increased steadily over 80 years

The incidence of multiple sclerosis appears to have been increasing in most countries of the world. It has been best studied in Canada where evidence suggests the disease has been increasing for some 80 years [162]. The increase has occurred more in women than men so that some three women now develop the disease for every man. The increase in multiple sclerosis and change in sex ratio cannot be explained by changes in diagnosis, changes in public awareness or anything of that kind [162]. Nor can smoking or use of the contraceptive pill explain the increase in women because the increase began before these social changes started.

One possible explanation of the greater increase of the disease in women that needs very serious examination is the difference between the two sexes in time spent out of doors during the teenage years and later. Teenage girls tend to give up sport and so spend much less time out of doors exposed to the sun than teenage boys who at the same age tend to be enthusiastic about outdoor activities. Low levels of vitamin D in teenage when the final growth spurt takes place. may cause errors in development of the growing nervous system. This difference between the sexes is now exacerbated by the inclusion of sun block in face creams and foundation make-up so reducing the small but important amount of vitamin D obtained by women through exposure of the face to the sun.

Dr Abhijit Chaudhuri became aware of Scotland's MS problem when he worked as a neurologist at Glasgow's Institute of Neurological Sciences, Govan Road. He tried unsuccessfully to persuade Health Boards in Orkney and Shetland to give vitamin D to schoolchildren. Now he works at the Queen's Hospital in Romford, Essex, where he recommends vitamin D to all early cases of MS.

Dr Chaudhuri said: "dietary supplementation of vitamin D in early life may reduce the incidence of MS. In addition, like folic acid, vitamin D supplementation should also be routinely recommended in pregnancy. Prevention of MS by modifying an important environmental factor (sunlight exposure and vitamin D level) offers a practical and cost-effective way to reduce the burden of the disease in future generations." [148]. Unfortunately at the time of writing the UK government's Healthy Start scheme, which is intended to be rolled out throughout the UK, is not working and children are not getting the extra vitamin D that they need for full health [93].

This failure of policy is very short-sighted since the financial cost alone, quite apart from the human misery, is immense. The cost of multiple sclerosis among the 466 million inhabitants of the European Union has been estimated to be around nine billion euros a year (this figure excludes Romania, Bulgaria and other countries joining the EU since 2005 but includes Iceland, Norway and Switzerland) [95]. Based on this figure, the cost to Scotland must be around 100 million euros annually.

Summary: Multiple sclerosis is more common in Scotland than anywhere else where it has been investigated. Much research on multiple sclerosis indicates that insufficient sunlight, and probably insufficient vitamin D is a cause of the disease. A proactive public health programme that increased the level of vitamin D in the population could be expected to reduce the incidence of the disease in Scotland.

2.2. Diabetes in young people (type 1) – a British record for Scotland

Scotland has a very high incidence of insulin dependent diabetes (diabetes type 1) surpassed only by Finland, Sweden and Sardinia. When a direct comparison of the different regions of the British Isles was last made in 1991 the incidence of diabetes type 1 in Scotland was found to be higher than in any other region [163]. This type of diabetes, often called juvenile diabetes in the past, blights young lives and despite modern treatments is plagued with complications that generally cause a premature death.

The incidence of diabetes type 1 in Scotland has been growing at a rate of 2% a year and reached 26.0/100,000 in children under 15 in 1993 [164]. The incidence in Aberdeen was separately found to be 26.4/100,000 in 1990-1999 [36]. This compares with an incidence of 17.7/100,000 for Oxford and 15.3/100,000 for Leicestershire in 1990-94 and in Yorkshire an incidence of 12/100,000 in 1978 rising to 20/100,000 in 2000 . The most recent results for Northern Ireland show an incidence of 22.3/100,000, intermediate between Scotland and England [165].

As in many other Western countries the incidence of diabetes type 1 has been increasing in Scotland for at least 30 years. The annual incidence in Europe increased by 3.4% annually between 1989 and 1994 with a higher increase among children less than five [166]. In some countries the increase appears to have reached a plateau but as yet there is no sign of this happening in Scotland [164]. Finland has an incidence of diabetes type 1 of 35/100,000 showing that a much higher incidence is possible; and the persistent increase in Scotland suggests that this level may well be reached if ways cannot be found to reduce risks.

The causes of this increase appear to lie, at least in part, in infant nutrition which has led to greater obesity and higher body mass index together with greater growth in height [5, 167-172]. The increases in height and weight of young people in many western countries over recent decades correlates well with the increase in incidence of diabetes type 1 over the same period. Taken together these correlations suggest that plentiful, and sometimes over generous, supply of food in childhood increases the risk of diabetes type 1 and is a cause of the increase in incidence. However other risk factors are involved too.

Several studies have found evidence that vitamin D supplements given to children can protect against diabetes type 1 [5, 166, 173]. A meta-analysis has calculated that supplementation with vitamin D may reduce the number of children developing diabetes type 1 by 30 per cent but higher doses and greater compliance might achieve a greater reduction [174].

North/south gradient

The suggestion that vitamin D insufficiency in early life is a factor in diabetes type 1 is backed up by geographical studies and studies of seasonal variation in the disease. In Europe a north/south gradient for the incidence of diabetes type 1 has been described [66, 175]. This gradient is what would be expected if exposure to sunlight and consequent synthesis of vitamin D were important risk factors for the disease. In Norway a reverse north/south gradient has also been described for serum vitamin D levels which can be explained by higher intake of fish (which is high in vitamin D) and supplements such as cod liver oil boosting vitamin D levels in certain regions [60].

Sardinia, an island in the Mediterranean, is a notable exception to the north/south gradient for diabetes type 1. This island has an incidence of diabetes type 1 of 37.8/100,000 which is four times that of nearby Lazio on the Italian mainland and almost the same as the incidence in Finland some 3,000 km to the north [165, 176]. Attempts to explain the high incidence of diabetes type 1 in Sardinia have concentrated on looking for genetic differences. However the high incidence could also be explained by differences in child rearing practices that do not yet seem to have been investigated in any detail. In some cultures women avoid the sun because they do not wish to develop a dark skin that is associated with lower social class and peasant status. Also in some societies mothers may remain largely indoors during pregnancy, a period still known as "confinement", and babies may be kept inside.

Such behaviour reduces exposure to the sun and vitamin D synthesis in the skin. The risk of diabetes type 1 in Sardinia has been found to be more closely associated with breast feeding than with bottle feeding which is consistent with what would be expected if the mothers had low levels of vitamin D [177]. Bottled milk is supplemented with vitamin D but breast milk is deficient in vitamin D when women have little exposure to the sun [178, 179].

Seasonal onset of disease

The date of onset of diabetes type 1 (taken as the first insulin injection) has been found to follow a seasonal pattern in Scotland with fewest new cases in the summer months (April to August inclusive) [164]. This pattern has been found in other European countries [165] and north America, and a similar summer dip has been found in the southern hemisphere [180, 181]. A summer increase in serum vitamin D is well documented [5] and, together with the seasonal evidence, suggests that vitamin D may, directly or indirectly, prevent emergence of the disease [5].

The seasonal cycle could also be triggered by infections that follow a well-known seasonal pattern. However it has been suggested that causality is in fact working in the opposite direction. Winter epidemics of influenza and other viral diseases may be the result of seasonal vitamin D insufficiency which reduces immunity and so increases the number of susceptible people in the population leading to outbreaks of disease [182].

We do not know whether the two recognised risk factors for diabetes type 1 discussed above, rapid growth of the baby and insufficient vitamin D, act together or independently in initiating the disease. However, from what we know of the action of vitamin D on cell growth and development it seems quite likely that they may act together. When cells in the pancreas are induced to grow rapidly with insufficient vitamin D they may not complete their normal development cycle and so remain immature. Such immature cells may trigger an autoimmune reaction that ends with the destruction of the insulin secreting cells. If this is the case then there is reason to hope that provision of vitamin D as a supplement in pregnancy and throughout childhood may very substantially reduce the incidence of diabetes type 1.

Mortality and morbidity of people with diabetes type 1 is very high and so even a modest percentage reduction in incidence of the disease would repay substantial dividends both human and financial [183]. People with diabetes type 1 have been shown to be at extra risk of suffering from fractures of the hip, confirming the high morbidity associated with diabetes and pointing to a common mechanism, vitamin D insufficiency, probably in early life [184].

Summary: Diabetes type 1 is very common in Scotland and increasing steadily in incidence. Bold action may be expected to reduce the incidence of the disease. All pregnant and nursing mothers should be given a supplement of 2,000 to 4,000 units of vitamin D a day and infants and children of all ages should also be given a vitamin D supplement. See discussion of supplementation for pregnant and nursing mothers: Westminster bungles supply of infant vitamins.

Diabetes in older people (type 2)

Vitamin D is now recognised to have an important role in controlling non-insulin dependent diabetes (type 2 diabetes) [185]. Observational studies show a relatively consistent association of low vitamin D status with type 2 diabetes and the associated condition, metabolic syndrome also known as syndrome X [5, 186-188]. The prevalence of diabetes is found to be about three times greater among people with low vitamin D levels compared with those who have high levels of the vitamin [185].

Diabetes type 2 is a major problem in Scotland but prevalence of the disease does not appear to differ significantly between England and Scotland [189]. The incidence of type 2 diabetes does not generally show a north/south gradient. Insufficient exercise and overweight are recognised as the major risk factors for type 2 diabetes but weight loss is difficult to achieve and maintain and exercise is difficult for people who are overweight and unfit. So other risk factors, such as the vitamin D level, which may be modified without undue effort of the subject, are important. Pittas *et al* conclude in their review and meta-analysis by remarking that "combined vitamin D and calcium supplementation may have a role in the prevention of type 2 diabetes especially in populations at risk of type 2 diabetes" [185].

Doctors at the University of Dundee.have begun to investigate this idea. They gave elderly patients with diabetes type 2, who lived on Tayside, a single large dose of vitamin D2 (100,000 IU) in a double blind randomised trial. The average serum 25 OH-D levels of the elderly diabetics moved into the normal range. They developed better function of blood vessels* and their systolic blood pressure decreased by 14mm of mercury [84].

Summary: Whether or not vitamin D and calcium play a part in prevention of type 2 diabetes, evidence suggests that they may be beneficial for people with the disease in optimising glucose and insulin levels following meals. So people with diabetes may be expected to gain a health benefit from measures taken to improve levels of vitamin D and calcium in the population as a whole.

2.3. Rheumatoid Arthritis – a northern affliction

Rheumatoid arthritis is a common condition in Scotland and it has been suggested that too little sunlight and insufficient vitamin D are probably risk factors for the disease [77, 119, 122, 149]. Rheumatoid arthritis not only causes crippling changes in joints but those who suffer from it have increased morbidity and mortality from cardiovascular disease and stroke brought about by acceleration of the atherogenic process that causes these diseases [190].

Low serum levels of vitamin D have been observed in patients with rheumatoid arthritis including newly diagnosed patients [191-194]. It seems likely that these low levels of vitamin D pre-date the disease and may be a contributory cause of it. Periods of high disease activity in patients with rheumatoid arthritis are associated with reduced levels of serum calcitriol, the active metabolite of vitamin D [195, 196].

Serum levels of vitamin D have also been found to be inversely related to the number of tender joints and other measures of intensity of symptoms in early rheumatoid arthritis [194]. Receptors for vitamin D have been found in cells in rheumatoid lesions including macrophages, chondrocytes, and synoviocytes but are absent in normal cartilage [197]. Progression of rheumatoid arthritis is associated with loss of bone mineral density, and low levels of vitamin D are likely to be a contributory cause of this [193, 198, 199].

Administration of vitamin D or its analogues to patients with rheumatoid arthritis has been found to reduce symptoms [196, 200-203] and has inhibited progression of artificially induced arthritis in mice [204]. Such evidence has encouraged rheumatologists to believe that vitamin D is an important risk factor for rheumatoid arthritis [205].

---

* Endothelial function as measured by flow mediated vasodilation of the brachial artery.

Environment more important than genes

A large population study of Danish twins found 13 identical twin pairs in which one twin had rheumatoid arthritis but no pairs in which both twins suffered from the disease. The Danish researchers concluded that genetic make-up is of minor importance in the development of rheumatoid arthritis [206]. This conclusion was disputed by researchers involved in genetic studies of the disease, but the Danish study remains the largest and most unbiased study available, based as it is on a large population sample. Differences in prevalence and incidence of rheumatoid arthritis in different countries and different areas must therefore be explained primarily by environmental risk factors.

A low prevalence of rheumatoid arthritis has been found in sunny regions including Pakistan [207], Africa [208], and in Hong Kong [209]. Rheumatoid arthritis is more common in northern than in southern Europe [194, 210-212] and seems to be less severe in patients in Greece and Italy than it is in British patients [213, 214]. Drosos et al found that 61% of British patients had more advanced disease compared with only 29% of Greek patients*. Drosos suggests that differences in sun exposure might account for the different clinical profile although other factors such as Mediterranean diet and genetic differences could also explain the observations [213].

A north/south gradient has also been found in the incidence of juvenile arthritis in Europe [215]. The highest incidence of the disease has been found in northern Norway (22.6 per 100,000) and Finland (18.2 per 100,000) with lowest rates in Germany (3.5 per 100,000) and France (1.3-1.8 per 100,000). Dr Boel Andersson Gare comments that these are probably true differences but uncertainty remains because different methods were used to obtain the figures [215].

The perceived benefit of a warm sunny climate has led Norwegian doctors to recommend treatment of rheumatoid arthritis and other diseases abroad in sunny lower latitudes paid for by the state [216].

High prevalence in Scotland

Prevalence of rheumatoid arthritis in Scotland seems to be among the highest known anywhere. Comparing figures from different studies is not easy because of differences in sampling methods, different definitions of disease, effect of age and relatively small numbers of people affected in samples of limited size [217]. Nevertheless prevalence of the disease in the Scottish Highlands is high. Average prevalence of the disease in Nairn, Black Isle, Lochaber and Skye was found to be 6.9 adults (over 15 years) per thousand [218].

A study based in Norfolk (England), which used different criteria, found a prevalence of 8.1 adults per thousand (women 11.6 per 1000, men 4.4 per thousand) [194]. This prevalence is about twice that found in Greece [213], or in northern Italy [210] or in Yugoslavia [219]. Prevalence of the disease in Dublin has been found to be 5 per 1000 comparable to that in Norfolk and Scotland [220]. The highest known prevalence of rheumatoid arthritis in the world, found in Rochester, Minnesota, is 14 per 1000 in women and 7.4 per thousand in men [221]. There appears to be little doubt that prevalence of rheumatoid arthritis in Scotland is high, but a detailed expert comparison of prevalence of the disease in Scotland with other locations would be valuable.

Prevalence in the Scottish Highlands was found to vary substantially between different locations. In the Black Isle 9.3 people per thousand were found to be affected by the disease compared with only 3.3 people per thousand on Skye [218]. Reasons for this were not explored but one obvious possibility is the amount of fish in the diet; fish being the best dietary source of vitamin D. The Black Isle is more of a suburban and farming community while Skye is more rural and more involved with fishing.

Dark skin carries high risk of rheumatoid arthritis

Scotland now has a substantial minority of Asians and other ethnic groups with darker skins. Dark skin may take up to five times longer to make the same amount of vitamin D as white skin [222, 223]. So it is worth noting here that experience of ethnic minority groups in the UK with rheumatoid arthritis is consistent with vitamin D insufficiency being the cause.

Rheumatoid arthritis is twice as common in Pakistani women living in England than in those living in their own country where the sun is much stronger [224, 225]. These women are at further risk because of cultural habits that demand the body be fully covered. Low back pain, a well recognised feature of vitamin D insufficiency is also more common in Pakistani women living in England than in those living in Pakistan [226]. These women are particularly at risk because they cover most of the body with clothing and so get very little exposure to the sun.

Unexplained musculoskeletal pain, frequently seen by GPs and rheumatologists, has been found to be common in South Asians and female asylum seekers in the UK and is associated with low serum levels of vitamin D and raised parathyroid hormone [227, 228]. However Black Caribbeans in Manchester have a lower prevalence of rheumatoid

---

* The study compared stage III or IV of radiological damage using the Steinbrocker classification.

arthritis compared with UK Caucasians and this may be explained by protection by greater exposure to sun in the West Indies during childhood and youth [229].

Rheumatoid arthritis has a high prevalence in the Faroe Islands that are located further north than Shetland at latitude 62°N. However, as in Mediterranean countries, rheumatoid arthritis in the Faroes appears to take a relatively mild course which has been attributed to the high fish diet of these islands [230]. A case control study in Seattle found that boiled or baked fish appeared to reduce the risk of rheumatoid arthritis [231] but there have also been negative findings for an association with fish [232].

Mediterranean diet or Mediterranean sun

Differences in manifestation of rheumatoid arthritis between northern and southern countries in Europe might be explained in part by diet as well as differences in sun exposure. A Mediterranean diet has been found to benefit patients with rheumatoid arthritis [233]. A study undertaken in Glasgow which provided cookery classes with instruction in Mediterranean cooking appeared to benefit women with rheumatoid arthritis. Fruit, vegetable and legume consumption increased and the women recorded improvements in pain score and early morning stiffness [234]. The Scots diet, which generally contains fewer vegetables, may be an additional risk factor for initiation of rheumatoid arthritis and/or may be a factor making symptoms worse.

Greater intake of vitamin D from food and/or supplements has been found to be associated with reduced risk of subsequent rheumatoid arthritis in the Iowa Women's Health Study [235]. However the Nurses Health Study found no association of dietary vitamin D and/or supplements with rheumatoid arthritis measured by questionnaire [236]. But the Nurses study made no measurement of sun exposure and so its negative finding lacks force. A prospective study of vitamin D in serum taken before development of the disease also had a negative finding, but an association could have been masked by difficulty in allowing for seasonal variation of vitamin D measurements [237]. Further studies are clearly needed to explore these associations in more systematic ways.

Fish and fish oils have been found in a number of studies to benefit patients with rheumatoid arthritis [238, 239]. These benefits have generally been attributed to the presence of omega-3 fatty acids in fish oils, although fish and certain fish oils are also an excellent dietary source of vitamin D. Studies using fish oil generally assume that omega-3 fatty acids are the active ingredient and neglect to note whether the fish oil preparation used contains vitamin D. In general fish liver oils are rich in vitamin D whereas fish body oils contain much less of the vitamin. Vitamin D content of fish and fish oil can also vary seasonally and certain preparations of purified omega-3 fatty acids have vitamin D removed. As a result it is impossible to know whether results obtained in studies using "fish oil" preparations may be influenced by the presence of vitamin D unless the issue is addressed explicitly.

Summary: There is much evidence, both direct and indirect, suggesting that insufficient vitamin D is an important contributory cause of rheumatoid arthritis. Prevalence of the disease is very high in the UK and low exposure to sunlight is almost certainly an important factor in the disease. Common mechanisms are involved in autoimmune disease and many features of rheumatoid arthritis show close parallels with both multiple sclerosis and diabetes type 1. Bradford Hill in his discussion of how to identify causes of disease from epidemiological observations suggests that analogy provides useful evidence for cause [128]. So, analogy with multiple sclerosis and diabetes type 1 adds force to the argument suggesting that insufficient vitamin D and/or sunlight is a cause of rheumatoid arthritis. And this leads on to the suggestion of practical measures that may be expected to reduce the risk of rheumatoid arthritis, e.g. taking of vitamin D supplements, especially in early life, and greater exposure to the sun.

2.4. Inflammatory bowel disease – silent suffering

Scotland is worse affected by Crohn's disease, an inflammatory disease of the bowel, than almost any country in the world. Only Denmark has more deaths per year from Crohn's. In Scotland annual deaths from Crohn's run at 4.65 per million of the general population compared with 3.43 in England suggesting a "Scottish effect" [240].

People suffer from Crohn's for many years often undergoing multiple operations, growth is stunted, distress is great and cost to the health service is very substantial. Prevalence of Crohn's is high because people live for a long time with the disease. An exact figure for prevalence of Crohn's in Scotland does not seem to be available but in England inflammatory bowel disease has a prevalence of about four per thousand people. About one third of these have Crohn's and the others ulcerative colitis [241, 242].

The incidence of Crohn's disease has increased steadily in Scotland since at least 1983, almost doubling over a period of 20 years. And the incidence in adults in Aberdeen has been found to be among the highest known anywhere in the world, reaching 11.6/100,000 in 1985-87 [243]. Over 30 years, between the late 1950s and the late 1980s, Crohn's disease increased some five fold in Aberdeen* and has begun to be found in children under 10 who never showed the disease previously [243].

This increase in incidence may be connected with a move away from a traditional diet rich in fish and hence in vitamin D to a relatively impoverished modern diet rich in refined carbohydrates. While Aberdeen has been Scotland's busiest fishing port for many years Aberdonians, like people everywhere, are likely to have changed their diet away from fish to a more universal international menu.

The Faroe islands have a very low incidence of Crohn's disease running at 1.75/100,000 in the 1980s, one-sixth of the incidence in Glasgow during the same period [245]. It seems likely that the reason for this may be a diet that remains closer to the traditional sea-fisher's diet than other regions of the north Atlantic seaboard, although Faroe islanders are now able to purchase all modern foods. The capital, Torshavn, now has a Burger King restaurant on the main street and it seems likely that changes in their diet may accelerate and vitamin D deficiency become more common.

Crohn's one of the most disabling chronic diseases

Scottish children appear to be more vulnerable to Crohn's disease than English children. In 1998-1999 the incidence in Scottish children under 16 was 4.2/100,000 compared with 3.1/100,000 for English children, suggesting again a "Scottish effect" [246]. Although the difference is not large it appears to have persisted over many years suggesting a real difference. In Scotland, Crohn's has been found to be significantly more frequent in children in the north of the country than in the south and to be more common in more affluent families and more common in urban than in rural areas [247].

Children with Crohn's disease suffer severely. In Scotland in the 1970s and 1980s children with the disease spent an average of nine weeks in hospital, many required surgery and a substantial proportion suffered stunting of growth [248]. While treatments have improved, Crohn's is still seen as one of the most disabling and disagreeable of all the chronic diseases.

Northern Europe and north America, where the sun is less intense and the summer season is shorter, have a higher incidence and prevalence of Crohn's disease than sunny southern regions, although rates are now rising in lower incidence areas such as southern Europe [243, 249]. Studies of veterans and the Medicare population in the United States have shown that inflammatory bowel disease, which is mostly Crohn's but also includes ulcerative colitis, is more frequent in the northern states [240].

The average mortality from Crohn's and ulcerative colitis, varies more than 60 fold in different countries round the world [240]. Some 60% of monozygotic twin pairs demonstrating Crohn's are discordant for the disease showing an important environmental contribution in causation of the disease. Furthermore the rapid increase in Crohn's in Scotland and elsewhere cannot be accounted for by genetics, which has dominated much research on this disease.

Low levels of vitamin D together with problems of osteoporosis and weak bones have commonly been noted in people with Crohn's [250-254]. Metabolic bone disease has been found to be present at diagnosis of Crohn's indicating that insufficient vitamin D is a condition of the disease at presentation and is not the result of drug treatments [251]. People with Crohn's also suffer from a high incidence of osteoporotic vertebral fractures [255].

Crohn's may sometimes occur as part of a more general "auto-immune syndrome". Inflammatory disease of the bowel has been found to occur together with multiple sclerosis in the same patient more often than would be expected by chance [256, 257]. Since both diseases involve inflammation and an autoimmune reaction it has been suggested that the two diseases may involve either a common process or common risk factors [257]. The finding of an increased incidence of focal lesions in the white matter of the brains of patients with inflammatory bowel disease also supports the suggestion that the disease may share a common mechanism of some kind with multiple sclerosis [258].

---

* Changes in diagnosis or increased awareness might account for this increase or some of it. However similar increases have occurred in other countries, for example Sweden, over the same time period suggesting that the increase is not an artefact. [244. See Lindberg, E., *et al.*, *Inflammatory bowel disease in children and adolescents in Sweden.* J Ped Gastroenterol and Nutr, 2000. **30**: p259-64.

D-deficient mice vulnerable to bowel disease

Psoriasis is also more common in patients with Crohn's disease and their relatives than in controls suggesting a link of some kind between proliferation and inflammation of skin and disordered growth of the gut lining found in Crohn's [259]. This link may well be vitamin D which has been shown to be beneficial in the treatment of psoriasis [260].

Crohn's disease, like multiple sclerosis, diabetes type 1, rheumatoid arthritis, and psoriasis is an autoimmune disease, and shares common epidemiological features with them. Low levels of vitamin D have been observed to be a feature of these diseases and it has been suggested that vitamin D status is likely to be important in prevention of these diseases [121]. This is supported by the observation that the active form of vitamin D has been shown to suppress the development of autoimmunity in experimental animals [261].

Margerita Cantorna and others have demonstrated a biological basis for inflammatory bowel disease with vitamin D insufficiency as a crucial risk factor. Animal experiments have shown how low vitamin D levels allow T cells to develop which may react against normal body tissues in an autoimmune fashion causing inflammatory bowel disease [120]. Furthermore vitamin D deficiency in mice has been shown to compromise the mucosal barrier of the gut leading to increased risk of inflammatory bowel disease in these animals [262, 263].

Infection, improvements in hygiene, antibiotics and use of refrigerators have all been suggested to play a part in causing Crohn's disease and its increasing incidence [249, 264, 265]. Infection certainly plays an important part in the disease itself but may be acquired after the disease has commenced.

Summary: Scotland has a high prevalence of Crohn's disease, among the highest known. The suggestion that insufficient vitamin D is a risk factor for the disease is supported by evidence of a north/south distribution in both Europe and north America, by low levels of vitamin D in the serum of patients who also have increased vulnerability to osteoporosis, multiple sclerosis, and psoriasis, and by a plausible biological mechanism supported by experiments with a model disease in mice. As with rheumatoid arthritis (see summary above) analogy with other autoimmune diseases such as multiple sclerosis and diabetes type 1 adds force to the suggestion that insufficient vitamin D and/or sunlight is a causal factor in the disease. A "Scottish effect" in Crohn's disease may be explained by the Scottish climate that provides less opportunity for exposure of skin to sun.

3. Asthma and other chest conditions

The prevalence of asthma in Scotland is among the highest in the world [266]. People in Scotland suffer more from wheezing, one of the main symptoms of asthma, than people in other parts of the UK [267, 268]. In Scotland 36.9% of people were found to suffer from wheezing during the previous year compared with 32.3% in England [267]. Asthma, it seems, may be another disease contributing to the Scottish effect.

The incidence of asthma has doubled in industrial nations since the 1970s [269]. According to a survey undertaken by Professor Graham Watt of the Department of General Practice in Glasgow University and others, prevalence of asthma in Renfrew and Paisley more than doubled in 20 years at the end of the last century [270]. Asthma is the commonest chronic disease of childhood in the UK. It occurs most frequently in cities and is least frequent in rural parts of third world countries. Rural children in Scotland are less vulnerable to asthma than their city cousins perhaps because they spend more time outdoors [271].

The disease commonly begins in children under six years of age suggesting that events in pregnancy or early life may be crucial. Following this lead, researchers in Aberdeen recorded the diets of 2,000 women in pregnancy and followed the children born subsequently to record the development of wheezing at ages three and five years. Professor Anthony Seaton and Dr Graham Devereux of the Department of Environmental and Occupational Medicine at the University of Aberdeen began by postulating that insufficient antioxidant vitamins (vitamin C and E) in pregnancy made the children more susceptible to inflammation of the airways by allergic substances.

Apples and fish

The Aberdeen team found that children who suffered from asthma, allergic sensitisation, wheeze and/or reduced lung function at the age of five were more likely to have a mother with low intake of vitamin E during pregnancy [272]. The children of these mothers with a low intake of vitamin E had symptoms of wheezing that were four times greater than those whose mothers had the highest intake (by comparison of highest and lowest quintiles of vitamin E consumption). Looking at the foods they ate, mothers who frequently ate apples or fish in pregnancy appeared to be protected from having children with poor respiratory symptoms [273]. The diet of the children themselves seemed to make no difference.

A similar study of 1194 mothers and their children undertaken by Scott T Weiss, Carlos Camargo and colleagues at Harvard Medical School in Boston, USA, found that mothers who obtained most vitamin D in their diet had a 40% lower risk of having a child with wheeze compared with mothers who obtained least vitamin D* [274]. The US researchers found that it made no difference whether vitamin D came from diet or from sunlight. Both were equally effective in reducing the risk of wheeze.

Vitamins D and E are both fat-soluble and intake of the two vitamins in food tends to be correlated. So the Aberdeen researchers looked again at their data in collaboration with the Harvard team and found that intake of vitamin D, as well as vitamin E, in pregnancy was a risk factor for wheeze in Scottish children. Thus confirming the basic observation of the US study [275].

However, further work from Carlos Camargo and others in Boston, USA, suggests that there is an important distinction between wheezing symptoms and true asthma [275.1]. They have shown that low levels of vitamin D found in blood taken at birth from the umbilical cord is associated with an increased risk of respiratory infections before three months and with wheezing later at 15 months, at three years and at five years. But low vitamin D in cord blood was not linked to an increased risk of asthma diagnosed by a doctor before the age of five. They concluded that higher levels of vitamin D in pregnancy may decrease the risk of early childhood wheeze by reducing respiratory infections, while some other factor is the cause of asthma.

Further research will be needed to find out if vitamin E is important. It may simply be carried along as a marker for vitamin D because both vitamins are fat-soluble. Already other studies support the suggestion that vitamin D has a beneficial effect on lung function. Men and women with the highest vitamin D levels in serum have been found to have better lung function** in an analysis of data from the Third National Health and Nutrition Survey (NHANES III) [276]. The difference was substantial, greater than that found between former smokers and non-smokers.

Other evidence from research not yet published in full appears to confirm the importance of vitamin D for normal lung function. A study of 2,112 adolescents has found that a low intake of vitamin D (157 IUs per day or less) is associated with poor lung function [277], and low serum vitamin D levels in children have been found to be associated with greater risks of severe exacerbations of asthma [278]. Experiments have also begun in giving vitamin D to people with asthma which is resistant to conventional treatment with steroids [279]. Vitamin D or its hormone form, calcitriol, has been shown to stimulate certain cells to produce a substance, IL-10, which inhibits production of irritating substances (cytokines) by cells that react to allergens. This is the first step in what may be a new treatment for asthma.

Where sea mists obscure the sun

Aberdonians, as we all know, traditionally eat a lot of fish because it is readily available and in the past it was also cheap. The extra vitamin D this provided must have been a great benefit to them since the climate on the east coast with its sea mists provides barely enough sun to give a satisfactory level of vitamin D. But eating habits have changed and the increase in asthma in Scotland in recent years may well be explained, at least in part, by a reduced consumption of fish as well as by reduced exposure to the sun.

In an enthusiastic editorial in the journal *Thorax* Scott T. Weiss and Augusto A Litonjua of Harvard Medical School and Brigham and Women's Hospital, Boston, wrote in 2008: "It seems likely that a gradual decrease in exposure to sun due to sun avoidance behaviours in Western societies (sunscreen, clothing, increased time spent indoors) reached a critical level in the early 1970s, such that humans were not spending enough time outdoors and vitamin D levels reached acutely low levels ... Vitamin D deficiency is the only factor that can explain all epidemiological aspects of the allergic and autoimmune disease epidemics noted above, and now the hypothesis that urgently needs testing is whether replenishment of pregnant women with vitamin D will have a major impact on the occurrence of all autoimmune diseases, particularly if it is followed by subsequent sufficiency of vitamin D in the developing child and adult." [269]

---

* by comparison of highest quartile of vitamin D uptake (median value of 724 IUs vitamin D per day) with lowest quartile (median value of 356 IUs).

** Shown by a higher lung capacity: a difference of 106 ml FEV1 – forced expiratory volume in the first second, and difference of 142 ml FVC – forced vital capacity. Comparison of top and bottom quintiles.

Breast versus bottle

It has been widely thought by paediatricians that breast-feeding would reduce the risk of allergies and asthma. However, surveys aimed at demonstrating such an effect have produced conflicting results. Some investigators have reported that breast-feeding protects against allergies while others have reported increased risks of allergy and asthma associated with breast-feeding. Differing results may be explained in part by methodological problems but also by differences in climate and available sunlight in the different parts of the world where these investigations have been made.

The methodological problems were addressed by Dr Malcolm Sears and colleagues in a survey of 1037 children born in Dunedin, New Zealand, in 1972/73 and published in The Lancet in 2002 [280]. Their hypothesis was that breast-feeding would protect against development of allergy and asthma in childhood. Dr Sears team found that children who are breast fed for at least a month, and for an average of 21 weeks, are more than twice as likely to suffer from asthma at age 9 than children who are bottle-fed. They concluded: "Breast-feeding does not protect children against atopy [allergy] and asthma and may even increase the risk".

However, a similar study of 2602 children born in sunny Perth, Western Australia, published in the British Medical Journal two years before came to the opposite conclusion. The BMJ summarised the findings in a "key message": "Exclusive breast feeding for at least 4 months is associated with a significant reduction in the risk of asthma and atopy [allergy] at age six years..." [281] Exclusive breast-feeding was also associated with reduced severity of asthma in two tropical countries: Kenya and Brazil [282, 283]. While, by contrast, a UK study found that only 2% of bottle-fed infants developed asthma compared with 4% of those breast-fed for one month or longer [284].

A study of some 500 children in Dundee found that breast feeding reduced respiratory infections up to age seven but made no difference to the development of medically diagnosed asthma [285]. However early introduction of solid feeding, before 15 weeks, was associated with an increased likelihood of wheezing being reported by parents. Solid feeding brings with it loss of the vitamin D supplement in bottle milk suggesting that insufficient vitamin D in months three and four of the babies life might account for the development of wheeze later.

A wide range of variables has been examined in these and other studies: early as opposed to late development of symptoms, wheezing as opposed to doctor diagnosed asthma, length of breast feeding, asthma in parents etc. Even so the conflicting results of the studies cannot be accounted for. One variable that has not been considered in any of these studies is supplementation with vitamin D, exposure to sunlight, or serum levels of vitamin D in mother and baby.

Breast milk varies in its vitamin D content depending on the exposure of the mother to the sun. This fact together with knowledge of the latitude where each infant feeding study was located may tell us something. Several studies that found a definite benefit of breast-feeding took place in sunny latitudes: Perth in Australia, Brazil and Kenya. While the two main studies with negative findings occurred in the UK and the south island of New Zealand where the sun is not strong enough in winter to produce much if any vitamin D. Sun exposure of mothers and babies and supplementation of the diet with vitamin D could be a key to understanding these findings and other studies of asthma and infant feeding which were located in Canada, Tucson, Arizona, and Italy – see references in [280].

Insufficient D driving the epidemic of chronic disease

The increase in the incidence or prevalence of wheezing or asthmatic symptoms has occurred in parallel with increases in the autoimmune diseases considered above: multiple sclerosis, type 1 diabetes and Crohn's disease. Asthma has similarities to these autoimmune diseases although it is not generally considered to be an autoimmune disease itself [286]. It appears that a common process, insufficient vitamin D, that is driving the increase in type 1 diabetes and multiple sclerosis may also be driving the increase in wheezing illness, if not true asthma.

Indeed the occurrence of diabetes type 1 and asthma in 16 European countries and 12 countries outside Europe is positively correlated [287]. However children who have diabetes type 1 and their siblings are less likely to suffer from asthma symptoms than other children [288]. This may be explained by vitamin D preferentially stimulating one or other of two immune responses (Th-1 or Th-2) that mutually inhibit each other [288].

A word of caution

An observation of wheezing, as recorded by the researchers in Aberdeen and Harvard, is not the same as a diagnosis of asthma and so there is uncertainty about the way these studies should be interpreted. Some of the children with wheeze may be suffering from inflammation of the chest following a virus infection rather than from persistent allergic asthma.

An alternative theory suggests that the epidemic of autoimmune disease and asthma is actually caused by too much vitamin D coming from fortification of foods such as margarine or, in the USA, milk [289-291]. It is difficult to see how a small quantity of vitamin D from foods that have been fortified since the 1930s or 1940s could be responsible for an increase in levels of disease occurring in the population during the latter half the 20th century. Fortification of foods may provide enough vitamin D to prevent most occurrences of rickets but they make only a small contribution to the final level of vitamin D in the population, which is in any case nowhere near what is considered to be optimal.

Nevertheless some evidence supports the theory. Doctors and scientists at the Medical Research Council Epidemiology Resource Centre in Southampton have found in a study of 596 pregnant women that mothers with highest serum levels of vitamin D in pregnancy were more likely to have a child with asthma than those with the lowest level of vitamin D [292]. However the numbers were small and the incidence of asthma in the children of women with high levels of vitamin D was the same as the national average. Therefore the finding could be an artificial result of the way in which information on asthma was collected.

In another study asthma and other allergic disease was found to be more frequent at age 14 and 31 years in members of the Northern Finnish Birth Cohort who were given a vitamin D supplement in the first year of life [293]. The infants were given a supplement of 2,000 IUs vitamin D per day, which is four times larger than supplements generally recommended for infants today.

Further research is needed to resolve these conflicting reports. This may be available soon if it is confirmed that severe exacerbations of asthma are associated with low levels of vitamin D [278]. This is an urgent matter for Scotland since respiratory disease is the third most common diagnosis of inpatient and day-case discharges and accounts for 8% of primary care prescribing [271].

Summary: It is not clear from the available evidence whether the risk of asthma might be reduced if mothers and babies increased their vitamin D intake; and it is not possible to interpret the studies of infant feeding and asthma adequately without information about the vitamin D uptake and/or serum levels of the mothers and babies involved. In general breast is best for prevention of infections and for healthy growth, but for prevention of chronic disease such as diabetes type 1 and multiple sclerosis breast-feeding mothers need to take a substantial vitamin D supplement. It seems likely that evolution will have determined an optimum uptake of vitamin D from all sources that will provide protection from all chronic disease including asthma. We are not sure yet what this is but it seems certain that most women fall way below it. Mothers in the UK who breast-feed for several months without taking a vitamin D supplement themselves and/or without giving their baby a supplement are putting the baby at risk of several chronic diseases, which may include asthma.

Chapter 4:
Bone disease, muscle disease and sport

1. Rickets and fractures in childhood

Children in Scotland appear to have weaker bones than children in southern England, another manifestation, it seems, of the "Scottish effect". Fractures in children are some 50% more common in Scotland and the north of England than they are in southern England* [294]. Weak bones are caused by insufficient vitamin D and/or calcium, which in extreme cases causes the classic bone disease, rickets. Less exposure to sunlight because of the Scottish climate is an obvious risk factor leading to weak bones that are more likely to break in accidents.

Children who suffer low energy fractures of the forearm have been found to have bones with a lower average density than other children [295, 296]. Studies following children from the womb to age nine years have shown that reduced density and strength of bones is associated with low levels of vitamin D in serum during late pregnancy [297-299]. Dr Jonathan Tobias of Bristol University and Dr Cyrus Cooper of Southampton University have argued on the basis of such evidence that bone development of adults is programmed by early life factors that may obviously include sunlight exposure and use of vitamin D supplements in pregnancy and early life.

Five infants on Tayside who were found to be suffering from rickets in 2007 reminded Scots that this is a problem that will not go away [300]. All five infants had been breast-fed and came from ethnic minority families. The risk of rickets is particularly great for breast-fed babies whose mothers have dark skin because the mother's vitamin D levels are particularly low during pregnancy and little vitamin D gets into breast milk [178, 179, 301-303]. Bottle fed babies rarely suffer from rickets because milk formula given to babies is nowadays supplemented with vitamin D. Mothers on a vegetarian diet, which is favoured by some Asian groups, also have an increased risk of D insufficiency and should not breast feed without taking a vitamin D supplement and giving a supplement to the baby [304].

Rickets was a serious problem in Scotland in the 19th and early 20th centuries, but disappeared in the 1940s because of fortification of margarine with vitamin D, free or cheap cod liver oil supplements provided by government for children from 1942, and the clean air acts passed in the 1950s which allowed more sunlight to penetrate city streets. But the problem re-appeared in Asians in Scotland in 1962 [305].

Asians in Glasgow

The risk of rickets in Asians living in the UK has been found to be greater the further north they live, supplying further evidence that the Scottish climate is in itself a risk factor for health. One in five Asian schoolchildren examined in Glasgow were found to suffer from low calcium in their blood or X-ray evidence of rickets compared with only one in ten in Coventry [90]. Rickets has also been recognised in other ethnic minority communities in England [306-308]. In winter 85% of Asians in Birmingham compared with only 3.3% of non-Asians had deficient serum levels of vitamin D (below 20nmol/L) [309].Clinical rickets is only found when children are grossly deficient in vitamin D, but for every child diagnosed with rickets the disease goes unrecognised in many more who suffer lesser distortions of the skeleton and weak bones together with increased risk of other chronic disease [308].

The importance of vitamin D for prevention of rickets and its role in growth of healthy bone has been known for almost 100 years. Vitamin D is now universally recognised to be essential for healthy growth in childhood. Supplements of vitamin D provide a complete cure of rickets and prevent the disease if given to babies. So the reappearance of rickets is a direct result of the failure in provision of vitamin drops to babies, both by the National Health Service Trusts and Boards in the regions and by central government in London.

Cod liver oil, which is the best natural source of vitamin D, was provided for children, either free or subsidised, by the government from 1942. In the 1970s cod liver oil was replaced by NHS infant vitamin drops containing vitamin D. But general uptake of the vitamin drops declined from the 1970s as successive governments progressively restricted free issue of the vitamins to families on benefits. This has put many children, regardless of race, at risk of poor bone development and growth as well as autoimmune disease (see Chapter 3).

Failure of Healthy Start programme to provide vitamin D

Recognising the problem, the UK government has now begun to provide new vitamin supplements containing

---

* 1988-98 figures for fractures in children aged up to 17 years corrected for differences in the age and sex structure of the population.

vitamin D to mothers and infants through the Healthy Start programme. However, this programme has up to now failed to deliver vitamin D supplements to most families in most parts of the country [93]. Provision of Healthy Start infant vitamins has been focused on children whose parents are on benefits despite the fact that vitamin D insufficiency is not caused by poverty but by lack of sunlight together with prolonged breast-feeding. Breast-feeding for six months or more should be the healthiest option for mother and baby but it cannot be recommended unless mothers and babies also take a substantial vitamin D supplement.

The Healthy Start programme is a UK national programme but responsibility for implementing it has been devolved to Health Trusts and Boards that in many areas have failed to get it going. For example Healthy Start infant vitamin drops have not been available in Edinburgh or on Tayside or in many parts of London. An energetic initiative by the Scottish government to provide pregnant women and infants with a vitamin D supplement could completely prevent rickets and at the same time reduce the risk of fractures in childhood and weak bones in later life. Great additional benefits in prevention of multiple sclerosis, diabetes type 1 and other autoimmune disease can also be expected by provision of these supplements (see Chapter 3) especially if an adequate supplement is continued throughout life.

In the late 1970s doctors in Glasgow showed that a successful public health programme could be organised that would increase uptake of vitamin D supplements by ethnic minority families [310]. Substantial efforts were made in Glasgow to deal with the problem but the initiative does not seem to have been taken up elsewhere in Scotland and eventually seems to have been lost. Nevertheless the Glasgow initiative shows that the problem can be solved without great expense if health professionals can be motivated.

Summary: Children in Scotland may be expected to grow up with weak bones unless they are given a vitamin D supplement. It has been known for 100 years that sunlight and cod liver oil are needed to make strong bones and that it is specially important for children to get sufficient vitamin D in the early years. But attempts of the present government to supply vitamin D to infants through the Healthy Start programme have been inconsistent and inadequate. This programme has been directed from Westminster but could be taken over and directed for Scotland from Edinburgh. See also: *Westminster bungles supply of infant vitamins*, Chapter 7, section 4.

2. Bone disease and adult fractures

Elderly patients in Scotland with fragility fractures have been found to have very low vitamin D levels. Nine out of 10 had a vitamin D level below 50nmol/L and the mean level was below 25 nmol/L. Gallacher *et al* from the Southern General Hospital in Glasgow conclude: "It may be that vitamin D represents a correctable risk factor for fragility fracture in the elderly" [4] . Elderly outpatients at the Victoria Infirmary, Glasgow, have also been found to have average levels of vitamin D that are insufficient for optimum health even though they were active and went outdoors regularly [6].

The incidence of limb and hip fractures has been found to follow a North/South gradient in Europe consistent with sunlight and vitamin D being a risk factor [311-313]. Sweden has the highest incidence of hip fracture in Europe followed by UK, the Netherlands and Germany, which have a similar hip fracture rate to the United States. While France, Greece and Spain have a rate about 70% of the United States; and Italy and Portugal have a rate 50% of the United States [312]. Older men and women with low levels of vitamin D are more vulnerable to fracture but the relationship is not strong suggesting that strength of bones may be determined for the large part earlier in life [314].

Hip fractures have also been found to be associated with diabetes, particularly diabetes type 1 which itself is linked to low levels of vitamin D in early life (see above) [184]. One prospective study failed to find any association between vitamin D levels in serum and subsequent fractures but such studies are difficult. A single blood sample is unreliable because seasonal variation in vitamin D levels obscures correlation with other factors [315].

The risk of fracture in Edinburgh men and women over 65 seems to be particularly high [316]. Comparison of incidence of fractures in Edinburgh and Dundee with England as a whole (represented by the General Practice Research Database - GPRD) suggests that fractures might be more frequent in the Scottish men in these cities than in the general English sample, but the comparison comes from different studies made at different times [316-318]. More detailed comparison of fractures in different age bands in Edinburgh and Dundee with Oxford and Leicestershire show that there is a great deal of overlap and a distinct pattern cannot be discerned [317]. While there is no clear evidence that Scottish adults are more at risk of fracture than their English cousins fractures are a universal problem that may be reduced if levels of vitamin D could be raised throughout life.

Hip fractures – low serum levels of vitamin D

Low levels of vitamin D in the body are associated with low absorption of calcium and increased bone turnover leading on to osteoporosis or osteomalacia (softening of bone) [319, 320]. A dietary survey of elderly patients with osteomalacia found that 50% had an intake of vitamin D less than 70 IU per day – that is less than five per cent of what might be considered a minimum intake necessary for good health [321].

Patients with hip fractures have average vitamin D levels in serum lower than those of controls [322, 323]. Some of these fracture patients have elevated parathyroid hormone (caused by low vitamin D) and they have been found to be at greater risk of injury to the heart around the time of their operation, suggesting that low vitamin D not only increases the risk of a fracture but also of a heart attack during the crisis period [324].

Serum vitamin D decreases during winter when a transient loss of bone density has been found to occur in women [325]. Advice from Cancer Research UK to reduce sun exposure in summer risks imposing an "artificial winter" leading to further reduction in vitamin D levels when these are already marginal. Such advice carries a risk of reducing bone density and increasing risk of fracture.

Several studies have found that supplementation of adults with vitamin D increases bone mineral density but improvement may not occur if there is not enough calcium in the diet [77]. For example, two randomised controlled trials have found that supplementation with either 800 IU vitamin D and 1200 mg calcium per day, or one capsule of 100,000 IU vitamin D every four months for five years, will reduce the risk of fractures [326, 327]. A meta-analysis of vitamin D supplementation concluded that daily doses of 700-800 IU or more decreased the risk of hip and other non-vertebral fractures whereas lower doses are ineffective [328]. However, discussion and review of evidence from these and other trials continue.

Conflicting results in vitamin D trials

At least five trials using various types of vitamin D supplementation have produced negative results for prevention of fractures [329]. Reasons for the failure of these trials to achieve high enough serum levels to prevent fracture include: use of the intra-muscular route which can be unreliable, use of vitamin D2 which may have reduced potency compared with vitamin D3, use of too small a dose in subjects who are severely depleted, poor absorption and/or poor processing in the liver and/or kidneys because of old age of subjects (75 years and over), and poor compliance – that is many people, particularly old people, forget to take their pills. In short these trials appear to have been foiled by the difficulty of raising vitamin D levels in old people who are severely depleted.

So, while some trials have found that a vitamin D supplement with or without calcium can reduce the fracture rate others have been unable to confirm it. To add to the confusion different meta-analyses, reviewing various sub-sets of trials, have come to differing conclusions [330-332]. For a comprehensive review of all relevant evidence and insight into the apparent discrepancies we must go to other sources [333, 334].

Tang and colleagues found that vitamin D did not offer additional risk reduction over and above the use of calcium alone [333]. They found some evidence for a beneficial effect of higher doses of vitamin D but their analysis was limited by the scarcity of data for vitamin D doses greater than 800 IUs per day. Tang *et al* conclude: "It is possible that vitamin D does have a beneficial effect when the dose is large enough (i.e. >800 IU). In the absence of such data, we recommend that if vitamin D is to be used as an adjunct supplementation to calcium, its dose should be at least 800 IU or more."

The possible beneficial effect of higher doses of vitamin D may perhaps be best understood when compliance to treatment and intake of any additional supplement are taken into account as shown by Bischoff-Ferrari in Figure 9. When this is done it may be seen that a serum level of vitamin D above about 75 nmol/L must be achieved for vitamin D treatment to be effective in prevention of hip fractures.

According to Bischoff-Ferrari a dose of 700 to 1000 IUs vitamin D per day will bring about 50% of adults over the 75 nmol/L level, while a dose of 4,000 IUs per day would be expected to bring 88% of younger adults of both sexes above 70nmol/L. However individuals with a lower starting level will require the larger doses, or more, if they are to reach the crucial 75nmol/L level [334]. Further support for Bischoff-Ferrari's interpretation comes from a trial of vitamin D and calcium supplement in naval recruits which has shown that 800 IUs per day of vitamin D plus 2000mg of calcium reduces the risk of stress fractures by 20% (see section 7 of this chapter for more details) [338].

Average levels of vitamin D are lower in Scotland than the United States and, as in any general population, many people who could potentially benefit will be older than those in these trials. This suggests that a dose of 4,000 IUs per day may be needed to bring the majority of Scots over the crucial 75nmol/L threshold that is most likely to be effective for reduction in risk of fractures. At present the maximum daily dose recommended in the UK is 1000 IUs and in the United States is 2,000 IUs. Doses up to 10,000 IUs per day have been found to be safe over several months

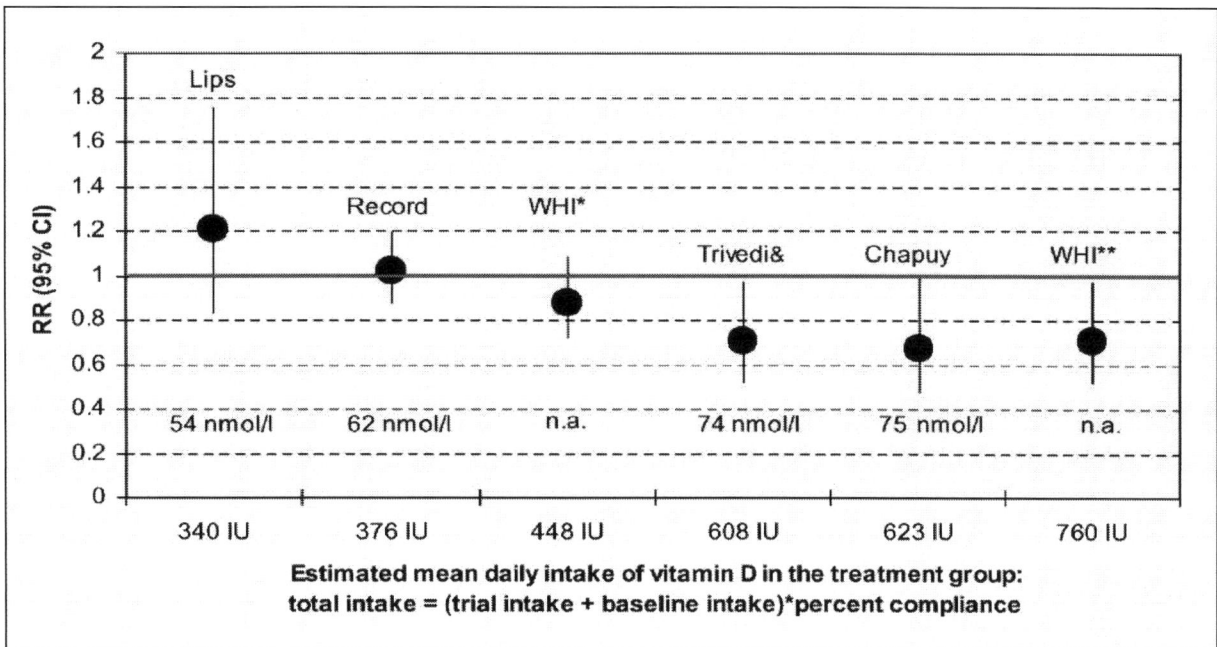

Figure 9. Results of trials of vitamin D in prevention of fractures can be understood when compliance with treatment and intake of additional vitamin D supplements is taken into account. The figure above is taken from Bischoff-Ferrari [334], who writes: "The graph suggests that efficacy increases with higher predicted actual mean intake of vitamin D in the treatment group. Studies that were successful in fracture reduction had an actual mean estimated intake of more than 600 IU per day, and associated achieved mean 25(OH)D levels were close to 75 nmol/l."

Details: Hip fracture efficacy by total estimated vitamin D intake (all trials used oral cholecalciferol) considering adherence to treatment. Compliance in the different trials was reported as follows: Lips (400 IU per day)=85% [335], Record (800 IU per day)=47% [336], WHI* intent-to-treat analysis (400 IU per day plus additional reported mean vitamin D intake of 360 IU)=59% [337], Trivedi (100,000 IU every 4 months equals 820 IU per day)=76% (&includes hip plus forearm fractures) [327], Chapuy (800 IU per day)=84% [326], WHI**-compliant women (400 IU per day plus additional reported mean vitamin D intake of 360 IU)=100% [337]. In most studies, being compliant was defined as taking 80% or more of the study medication. The x-axis gives the DiaSorin equivalent 25(OH)D levels in nmol/l achieved in the treatment arm of the trials. #For the Record trial a HPLC method has been used for 25(OH)D measurement with an unknown DiaSorin equivalent value. In the WHI trial, 25(OH)D levels have not been measured at follow-up in the study population (n.a. = not available)

[339] but there is a small risk of hypercalcaemia and so trials will be needed before doses above 2,000 IUs can be recommended for the population at large.

Since compliance has been identified as a major problem it makes sense to consider providing vitamin D to individuals by multiple routes. Bischoff-Ferrari suggests that adherence might be improved using sunbed exposures and that an annual intra-muscular injection with 300,000 IUs vitamin D together with a daily supplement might be a useful approach in clinical practice. Use of multiple routes is more likely to achieve high serum levels, especially in older people whose absorption or skin synthesis of vitamin D is limited. These trials show that it is not easy to repair lifelong damage caused by too little vitamin D by giving supplements in old age. Despite the negative findings of some trials there can be little doubt that insufficient vitamin D is a major cause of weak bones and that supplements can be beneficial, as shown by the benefits in preventing stress fractures [338].

The UK's distinguished Standing Scientific Committee on Nutrition (SACN) has reviewed the trials of vitamin D for prevention of fractures [158] but overlooked the importance of achieving a threshold blood level before benefit is obtained. Professor Reinhold Vieth, Canadian expert on vitamin D from the University of Toronto, commented: "In the context of clinical trials, the SACN focused on two large UK trials reported in 2005, Grant *et al* and Porthouse *et al*, that failed to demonstrate fracture prevention. Despite acknowledging the shortcomings of those trials, the SACN ignored the evidence from fracture prevention trials that showed positive results require serum vitamin D greater than 72 nmol/L." [339].

Fractures – a major cause of death

Osteoporosis and other bone diseases are a major cause of morbidity and mortality. Almost half the UK population has experienced a fracture of some kind in their lifetime [340]. Some 40% of women and 13% of men suffer fractures of the spine, hip or wrist that are made more likely by osteoporosis. Between 10 and 20% of people die within six months of a hip fracture and 50% of those who have suffered a hip fracture are unable to walk again without assistance.

The annual cost of osteoporosis in the USA has been estimated to be $5-10 billion with a similar pro rata cost in other developed countries [341]. In the UK the cost of hip fractures alone has been put at between £726 million and £1.7 billion per year [342, 343].

The benefit from vitamin D in enabling growth of healthy bones is enough in itself to favour a public health policy that recommends safe sunbathing – sunlight being our major source of vitamin D. An eminent panel of doctors and scientists concerned with bone disease called for a review of UK public health programmes on sunlight as long ago as 1998. Their report, Nutrition and Bone Health [3], recommended that "the public health consequences of sunlight exposure should be reviewed to take account of both its beneficial and its adverse effects with a view to developing guidelines. The effect on vitamin D status of measures taken to reduce the risk of skin cancer, such as encouraging covering up with clothes and applying cosmetic creams which seek to prevent the UVR reaching the skin should be clarified." This recommendation was never taken up and is now more urgent than ever.

Summary: Fractures are a major cost to the health service and a major cause of death and disability in Scotland as elsewhere. Trials suggest that falls and fractures can be prevented if sufficiently large doses of vitamin D3 are given. At present government does not recommend any vitamin D supplement for healthy adults in the UK. The United States and Canada both recommend a vitamin D supplement for healthy adults. This advice needs to be reviewed by Scots experts with the special needs and priorities of Scotland in mind.

3. Dental decay – more to it than fluoride

A consistent north/south variation in the prevalence of dental caries has been found in the UK. Children from Scotland, the Northwest, Wales and Mersey regions have consistently been found to have more caries than children in the south of England according to studies made by the British Association for the Study of Community Dentistry [344].

The proportion of 12-year-old children with untreated dental caries was three times greater in Scotland than in the South West Thames region in 1991/2. While 55% of Scottish five year olds in 2003/4 had evidence of caries invasion of dentine compared with only 40% of English five year olds [344]. In 2005/6 Scottish five year olds showed some improvement but their teeth remained substantially worse than those of English children of the same age [344]. There could be many reasons for these differences including differences in diet, poverty, and softness or hardness of the water supply. But differences in exposure to sunlight and vitamin D levels could also account for some of the differences in tooth decay between north and south Britain.

There was a time when the teeth of Scots children on the Hebridean island of Lewis were the envy of Britain. A district nurse on Lewis is quoted as saying early in the 20th century: "the most striking fact in the adult population [of Lewis] is their beautiful teeth" (Carnegie Trust's Report on the Physical Welfare of Mothers and Children in Scotland, 1913, quoted by King [345]). A survey undertaken in the 1930s found that in one district of Lewis some 50% of children were found to be entirely free of caries compared with only 6.3% in West Ross-shire, 1.9% in London and 2.5% in Sheffield during the same period [345]. The survey found that these island children were eating about half a pound (about 225 gm) of fish a day, providing about 1500 IUs of vitamin D. Children on the island living an urban life in Stornaway and eating fish less frequently had a much higher incidence of caries, similar to those in West Ross-shire.

The importance of vitamin D for healthy development of the teeth was established by M. Mellanby in the 1920s and 1930s – for references see King [345]. In 1936 the Dental Disease Committee of the Medical Research Council concluded: "The investigations described in this report show conclusively that a relatively high vitamin D content of the food can do much to diminish the incidence of caries if the vitamin is given during the development of the teeth; that a beneficial effect may be obtained if the vitamin is given at a fairly late stage of development; and that even when it is given after the eruption of the teeth, the onset and spread of caries is delayed."

The relationship between sunlight and prevalence of tooth decay was understood about the same time and demonstrated in a study of data obtained by the US Public Health Service in 1939. A clear relationship was shown between prevalence of tooth decay and hours of sunshine in an analysis of the teeth of white boys living in small communities [346]. Boys living in the sunny southern states had an average of about three cavities each compared with five cavities each for boys living in the least sunny northern states.

Faults in enamel

The teeth are made from deposits of a dense calcium containing material. Since vitamin D is central to the body's control of calcium absorption and metabolism, it is not surprising to find that deficiency of vitamin D and sunlight have a role in dental decay (caries). The formation of dentine (the solid material in teeth) begins in the last two months of pregnancy and continues until eight or nine years of age, while the wisdom teeth (third molars) continue to form during the following 10 years [308]. So exposure to sunlight during pregnancy and throughout childhood, together with vitamin D in the diet or in supplements, may be expected to be important for the formation of strong teeth. The teeth are completed with the laying down of enamel, an insoluble calcium phosphate compound.

Delayed eruption of teeth and hypoplasia (faulty development) of the dental enamel are recognised as signs of rickets [308]. Supplementation of mothers with vitamin D during pregnancy has been shown to prevent hypoplasia of the enamel in infants which may occur without other symptoms of rickets [347, 348]. Hypoplasia of the dental enamel has been found to occur more frequently in low birth weight babies born in winter or early spring months when vitamin D levels in the body are lowest [349]. This is consistent with sunlight and vitamin D being important for sound development of teeth. Enamel hypoplasia allows carious lesions to become established more easily, making people vulnerable to other dietary factors which increase the risk of caries.

Vitamin D is also important for the health of teeth in old age. A randomised, placebo controlled trial has shown that tooth loss can be prevented in old people by vitamin D [350]. Supplements of vitamin D (700 IU) and calcium (500 mg) were given to 145 people over 65 years of age. Those taking supplements were found to have lost half as many teeth as those taking placebo when assessed 18 months after the start of the trial. It appears that deficiency of vitamin D allows softening of the bone in the jaw with loosening and consequent loss of teeth.

Periodontal disease has also been associated with low bone mineral density (osteoporosis) and insufficient vitamin D [350, 351]. Furthermore periodontal disease itself has been associated in the Health Professionals Follow-up Study with an increased risk of cancer, particularly lung, kidney, pancreas and blood (haematological) cancers [352]. The authors suggest that periodontal disease might be a marker for a "susceptible immune system" which makes a person vulnerable to cancer. Indeed a susceptible immune system may be induced by insufficient vitamin D, which we know is a common risk factor for all three diseases: periodontal disease, osteoporosis and cancer. Optimists have suggested that improved oral hygiene, i.e. brushing and flossing, may prevent cancer. While periodontal disease is likely to benefit from such attention it seems too much to hope that it may prevent cancer. More to the point, periodontal disease may be seen as a sign of failing immunity that may eventually have devastating consequences elsewhere in the body if it is not treated by taking a suitable vitamin D supplement.

Summary: There can be little doubt that an adequate level of vitamin D will aid development of strong gums and healthy teeth. The importance of dietary calcium, vitamin D and sunlight for good development of teeth appears to have been generally overlooked. Emphasis has been given in public health campaigns to the effects of diet, fluoride, and tooth brushing in preventing tooth decay. Sunlight and vitamin D uptake also appear to be important and need to be recognised in public health policy, particularly in Scotland where sunlight is in short supply.

4. Unexplained backache and muscle pains

Insufficient vitamin D may not only weaken bones but it may also cause muscle weakness, muscle pains, and body sway which are a contributory cause of falls [224, 353, 354]. Muscle strength has been found to be correlated with serum vitamin D levels in old people [355]. Levels of vitamin D below 50 nmol/l are associated with sway and below 30 nmol/l with decreased muscle strength [353, 354]. Supplementation with vitamin D for 1 to 2 months has been shown to normalise muscle strength in patients with myopathy [356, 357] and supplementation with vitamin D plus calcium has been found to reduce falls in the elderly [62, 358].

People with darker skin and older people who seldom get out of the house suffer frequently from unexplained musculoskeletal pains, particularly back pain [225]. This type of pain seems to have increased between two and four fold in the north west of England over the last 40 years and the increase may possibly be accounted for by changes in habits of exposure to the sun providing lower levels of vitamin D [208]. Pains of this type are a recognised symptom of osteomalacia which is readily diagnosed by tests for calcium, vitamin D and parathyroid hormone in serum [227, 228, 359, 360]. However these patients are typically seen by rheumatologists and other specialists who generally do not appear to include hypovitaminosis D in the differential diagnosis of bone pain.

A Dutch study in 1996 found that it took on average almost five years for a diagnosis of hypovitaminosis D to be established in such cases [361], and a Swiss study in 2004 found that it took an average of three years [228]. There is no reason to believe that the delay in diagnosis of such cases is much different in the UK today.

While writing this I was contacted by an Indian doctor, an anaesthetist working in Northern Ireland, who suffered severe pains for 10 years before osteomalacia was diagnosed. During these 10 years he also suffered from tuberculosis and consulted numerous different doctors from a wide range of specialties, none of whom tested him for vitamin D deficiency. Finally a young physician he had not consulted before noticed his calcium was low and finally a vitamin D test was obtained.

After more than 12 months of vitamin D treatment, 12 years after the start of his pains, the doctor's vitamin D level had increased to a satisfactory level, but he still suffered from painful muscle weakness (myopathy), a consequence of his osteomalacia, and was unable to rise easily from a chair without help. Finally he started sun-bathing on a holiday to India. His pains diminished considerably and he felt significantly stronger. One case of course proves nothing, but it is consistent with the results of research and illustrates the problem.

Once doctors start to look out for osteomalacia and hypovitaminosis D the problem is found to be common. One study found that 78% of Indo-Asian patients attending a UK rheumatology clinic suffered from hypovitaminosis D compared with 58% of controls [222]. Dr Helga Rhein, an Edinburgh GP, tested 99 of her patients, aged 15 to 85, who she suspected of having vitamin D deficiency [362]. About half were South Asian or belonged to some other ethnic minority. Many of the patients complained of vague musculo-skeletal symptoms, were overweight, house bound or for some other reason had little exposure to sunlight.

Only two per cent of Dr Rhein's patients had a satisfactory vitamin D level. The rest, including all the ethnic minority patients she tested, had levels of vitamin D generally regarded as insufficient and almost half had levels that were frankly deficient (below 25 nmol/L). Symptoms in such cases may disappear after one to seven months treatment with two intra-muscular injections of vitamin D (300,000 IUs) and 800 IUs vitamin D per day orally [228]. Larger daily doses of vitamin D3 up to 4,000 IUs per day are increasingly being prescribed in other countries, but suitable preparations providing higher doses are not available in the UK as a normal part of the doctors list of prescribable drugs.

Summary: Many people are suffering needlessly from back pain and other muscle pain caused by low vitamin D. Low back pain alone costs £12 billion a year in the UK [363]. Raising levels of vitamin D in the population can be expected to do much to reduce unexplained back and other muscle pains.

5. Muscle weakness and depression

Vitamin D supplements are necessary to maintain muscle strength, balance and stability and prevent falls in old people who have insufficient levels of the vitamin [328, 353, 354, 360, 364, 365]. Speed of walking, ability to rise quickly from a chair, and handgrip strength are associated with vitamin D levels in old people [366, 367]. Reduced levels of vitamin D and increased levels of parathyroid hormone (which increases as D decreases) have been found to be associated with depression in elderly people and hyperparathyroidism is well known to be associated with depressive symptoms [368]. A large trial is necessary to prove whether a vitamin D supplement will alleviate depression but evidence as it is now suggests that vitamin D may be a very effective tonic for the elderly providing a range of benefits.

Young people may also be weak as a result of vitamin D insufficiency. Schoolgirls in the Lebanon increased their lean muscle mass when given a vitamin D supplement of 2000 IU/day [369].

The implications of these observations for maintaining the health and independence of old people are immense. However trials have shown that it is not easy to supplement old people with vitamin D because of problems of compliance (especially when vitamin D is provided with calcium), problems of absorption, and problems of providing a sufficient dose to obtain a significant rise in serum levels [334, 336]. It may be that exposure to UVB from the sun or sunlamps is a more effective way of boosting levels in old people and further work needs to be done on this [370].

Summary: Low levels of vitamin D in Scottish people, especially in winter, are a major cause of muscle weakness and hence tiredness. Boosting vitamin D levels in the general population can be expected to improve general strength, fitness and well being and reduce the incidence of fractures in old people caused by falls.

6. Sport – is Scotland achieving its potential?

A high level of vitamin D is essential for optimum muscle action and can make a vital contribution to peak athletic achievement [371]. Scottish athletes are at a disadvantage living in a climate which provides them with little sunlight and little vitamin D, a climate which gives the average Scot insufficient vitamin D in summer as well as winter [5]. Even in a sunny climate athletes who train mainly indoors can have an inadequate level of vitamin D. Elite gymnasts in Australia have been found to have sub-optimal levels of vitamin D that might be expected to affect their performance [372].

Scottish sportsmen and women may be prevented from achieving their true athletic potential if, like most Scots, they have low levels of vitamin D in their bodies. Astonishingly this issue does not seem to have been investigated in Scotland, or, indeed in England. In southern England up to 50% more sun is available in the active UV range for making vitamin D compared with Scotland [373]. This is enough to make a significant difference in vitamin D levels between the two countries and could affect sporting achievement [24].

A seasonal variation in muscular strength and fitness has been documented in athletes and pilots [374]. Some athletes notice a dip in performance in winter that does not begin to improve much until April or May when at last the sun is strong enough to provide some vitamin D. As the Scottish proverb goes: "Ne'er cast a clout 'til May be oot". It is not until May that it is generally warm enough in Scotland to remove some clothes and expose more skin to the sun. Anyone, athlete or not, experiencing a marked winter dip in fitness is well advised to consider whether vitamin D insufficiency may be involved and to take a vitamin D supplement.

Evidence buried in old research

Scottish athletes compete internationally with others who have trained in the sun. Scottish football teams play Spanish, Italian and other teams that have the opportunity to be exposed to much more sun than they are. It is possible that Scottish sportsmen and women might achieve better results internationally if they took a regular vitamin D supplement. This is especially important for athletes who play or train indoors such as swimmers, and competitors in basketball, squash, fencing and other indoor activities because they obviously obtain less exposure to the sun during the normal course of their training.

Muscle weakness in old people with low levels of vitamin D is well known to researchers ([354] and more references above); but few scientists and sportsmen outside the former Iron Curtain countries understood, at least until quite recently, that a good level of vitamin D is also necessary for achieving maximum fitness in sport. Scientific evidence on vitamin D and sports fitness remained buried in old German and Russian literature until Dr John Cannell, founder of the Vitamin D Council and veteran researcher in the subject, dug it out.*

Much groundwork on vitamin D and sporting fitness was done in Germany in the 1920s and later. Interest in the virtues of sunlight chimed with the increasingly popular belief in healthy outdoor pursuits such as hiking. And in the 1930s German sports scientists knew they could count on the support of Hitler who was doing everything he could to prepare for success in the Berlin Olympics in 1936. The following summary from a German journal translated by Dr Cannell and colleagues shows how far ahead German sports scientists were between the wars.

"It is a well known fact that physical performance can be increased through ultra-violet radiation. In 1927, a heated argument arose after the decision by the German Swimmers' Association to use the sunlamp as an artificial aid, constituting an athletic unfairness, doping, so to speak. In 1926, Rancken had already reported the improving effect of sunlamp irradiation in swimming times after repeated irradiations. In thorough experiments, Backmund showed that a substantial increase in muscle activity happens after radiation of larger portions of the body with an artificial sunlamp; that this performance increase is not caused through local – direct or indirect – effects on musculature, but through a general effect. This general effect, triggered by ultra-violet irradiation, is caused by a systematic effect on the nervous system [375]."

UV radiation knocked seconds off 100m dash

In 1952 Spellerberg, a sports medicine researcher in Germany, reported further experiments showing improvements in athletic performance after irradiation with a UV lamp. The results were sufficiently impressive for the Sports College of Cologne to officially notify the "national German and international Olympic committee".

Meanwhile behind the Iron Curtain, in the heyday of the communist empire, athletes, trainers and their medical advisers were under great pressure to produce sporting results that reflected the greatness of Marxism-

---

*I am deeply indebted to Dr Cannell in what follows in this section. Without his painstaking research in old journals and the lively presentation in his newsletter this work would not have come to light.

Leninism. In 1938 Russian sports scientists showed that college students who underwent a course of UV irradiation as part of training were able to knock a second off their average time in the 100m dash [376]. Students not given the irradiation improved by only two-tenths of a second. And so the Russians pushed their athletes hard, encouraged them to top up their vitamin D, and won many medals in the 1960s and 70s.

A number of other researchers have reported benefits from using sunlamps and boosting vitamin D including: improved athletic performance, improved cardiovascular fitness, better muscular endurance, improved muscle strength, reduction in resting pulse and improved reaction times [374]. Other experiments have shown that taking vitamin D supplements can actually increase muscle mass and increase the number of "fast twitch" fibres that are crucial to athletic performance, at least in people who are not getting enough vitamin D in the first place [374].

A recent review entitled *Should we be concerned about the vitamin D status of athletes?* concluded: "... it is likely that compromised vitamin D status can affect an athlete's overall health and ability to train (i.e. by affecting bone health, innate immunity, and exercise-related immunity and inflammation). Although further research in this area is needed, it is important that sports nutritionists assess vitamin D (as well as calcium) intake and make appropriate recommendations that will help athletes achieve vitamin D status: serum 25(OH)D of at least 75 or 80 nmol/L." This review provides much useful detail for those advising athletes on their health [377].

Summary: Low levels of vitamin D impair optimum function of the nervous system, muscles and other body process-es. Sports doctors in Russia and East Germany have known about this for many years. Astonishingly this knowledge has been completely overlooked in the West where athletes, like everybody else, have been told to avoid sun exposure for fear of skin cancer, so lowering their vitamin D and most likely their performance too. All Scottish athletes would be well advised to take a supplement of 2,000 IUs vitamin D per day (or equivalent dose weekly or monthly) and to train in a sunny climate for several weeks a year, especially in winter, if this is possible. Careful sunbathing, exposing as much of the skin as possible without using suncream while taking care not to burn, is a safe way to raise vitamin D levels.

7. Sport – stress fractures

Stress fractures are common in military recruits doing basic training and in athletes at all levels of training. Taking calcium and vitamin D can substantially reduce the risk of these fractures.

A stress fracture is a partial or complete bone fracture that is the result of a repeated stress that is not sufficient to cause damage when applied just once. Stress fractures occur when bones are repeatedly loaded over short periods without time for repair. These fractures are recognised initially by the occurrence of local bone pain that increases with weight bearing or by repeated use. Continuous pain lasting over three weeks is a warning sign suggesting a stress fracture. Standard X-rays generally do not show any damage. To confirm diagnosis a nuclear magnetic resonance scan or triple phase nuclear medicine bone scan is needed.

Runners, tennis, basketball, and football players, and ballet dancers are all at risk. The shaft of the tibia/fibula are common sites to be affected in most athletes, but basketball players often experience stress fractures of the malleolus (ankle bones) and the metatarsals (feet), while track, field and soccer players are at risk of fracturing the pubic bone, and rowers of fracturing a rib.

A survey of university of California division 1 athletes found that 6% of 6900 athletes followed over 14 years experienced a stress fracture of some kind but higher rates of 10 to 31% have been found in track and field teams [338, 378]. Typically an athlete must rest or reduce activity for six to eight weeks when a stress fracture occurs before returning to their sport. Stress fractures are common in military recruits with fracture rates for males ranging from 0.2 to 5.2% and for females from 1.6 to 21.0% [338]. Stress fractures have cost the US army millions of dollars for medical expenses of invalided personnel. Furthermore about half those personnel who experience a stress fracture do not complete military training and have to be discharged.

A trial to test whether calcium and vitamin D could prevent fractures followed 3700 naval recruits for eight weeks at the Great Lakes Naval Training Centre in Illinois. Of these 309 (5.9%) women suffered 496 stress fractures, mostly of the tibia and fibula. The fracture rate was reduced by 20% in women navy recruits who took a supplement of calcium (2000 mg per day) and vitamin D (800 IU per day) [338]. The dose of vitamin D used in this trial is not large; so a further reduction in stress fractures may be expected with higher doses of vitamin D.

High levels of physical activity cause considerable loss of calcium in sweat. If a person sweats heavily and is taking in insufficient calcium this results in additional stress to the skeleton because the shortfall in calcium must be mobilised from the bones. A single bout of moderate endurance exercise can cause increased turnover of bone that limits its ability to repair stressed regions. An elite athlete can lose as much as 20% of his or her leg bone mass in the course of an annual season of sport.

Loss of calcium was measured in 11 members of the University of Memphis basketball team by Klesges *et al* [379] who found that leg bone mass decreased by 6% over a period of four months. Players lost on average 422 mg of calcium during a single two-hour training session. Supplementation with calcium and vitamin D (using doses tailored to estimated individual losses) increased their leg calcium by 3% over a period of four months.

Summary: Recruits and athletes who have low levels of vitamin D and/or high levels of parathyroid hormone have been found to be more vulnerable to stress fractures. Supplementation with calcium and vitamin D can reduce fractures and minimise failure of individuals in competitive sports. It can also prevent failure of training in the forces. Supplementation may enable substantial saving of money in the forces and in professional sports.

Chapter 5:
Winter illness and other infections – need we suffer so much flu and so many colds?

1. Dramatic effect of D on immune system

Vitamin D deficiency increases the risk of tuberculosis [380, 381] and probably increases the risk of virus infections, in particular influenza [182], colds [382] and shingles [383]. The sunshine vitamin has a dramatic effect on the immune system that enables it to fight infection without the pains and malaise that are associated with a severe immune response and the worst aspects of flu.

Optimal levels of vitamin D in the body enable the production of anti-microbial peptides which play a major part in protecting the lung against infection [384]. Vitamin D also modulates the activity of the immune system preventing excessive production of cytokines which cause inflammation and the extreme malaise that generally accompanies influenza [385]. So a person with optimal levels of vitamin D should be less likely to develop flu or colds but if they do the symptoms may be expected to be considerably milder. A study of young men in the Finnish military has found that those with lower levels of vitamin D have more days of absence from duty because of respiratory infections [386].

Respiratory diseases, including influenza and colds, occur most frequently in Europe and north America in winter with a peak of incidence in December to March when vitamin D levels are at their lowest. In the southern hemisphere they occur in the corresponding winter months. Unfortunately comparison of the incidence of influenza in Scotland and England cannot be made easily because different definitions are used to record the flu-like illness north and south of the border.

2. Tuberculosis: more common in spring

Respiratory syncitial virus is the most important respiratory pathogen in early life, causing many infants to be hospitalised. Timing of occurrence of epidemics of respiratory syncitial virus has been studied round the world. Activity of the virus has been found to be inversely proportional to available UVB from sunlight at three locations in temperate climates, suggesting that vitamin D levels probably play an important part in epidemics of this virus. In tropical and sub-tropical locations epidemics tend to occur in the rainy season when cloud reduces UVB radiation [387].

Tuberculosis is more commonly notified in the UK in late spring or early summer than at other times of year [388]. It appears that the infection is most likely to begin spreading when vitamin D levels are lowest in February or March and reaches a stage when illness becomes severe and diagnosis is made in April or May. This seasonal pattern occurs mostly among migrants from the Asian subcontinent, who are particularly subject to vitamin D deficiency in the UK; whereas the occurrence of the disease among whites occurs more evenly throughout the year [389].

Asian immigrants to the UK have a relatively high incidence of TB probably because they bring dormant infection with them. The dormant infection is then activated by deficiency of vitamin D caused by low exposure to sunlight in the UK compared with their country of origin and low absorption of UV by dark skin [77, 380]. The disease is most likely to be activated in January when vitamin D levels are lowest but does not reach a stage where it can be recognised clinically until late spring or early summer.

As well as evidence from the influence of the seasons, there is interesting geographical evidence for the influence of sun exposure in prevention of TB. The incidence of tuberculosis in regions of Spain correlates closely with the annual hours of sunshine [390]. In the Bajo-Deba valley region of the Basque country very different incidence rates were observed in neighbouring towns with similar levels of income and education. Over a period of eight years the incidence in the two inland towns, Ermua-Mallabria and Mendaro, was 95.6 per 100,000 inhabitants in contrast with 26 per 100,000 for two nearby coastal towns, Deba and Mutriku. The two inland towns are located in narrow valleys that are colder and receive less sun than the two towns on the coast. Average serum levels of vitamin D in a random sample of pregnant women in the coastal towns were much greater than in the inland valleys (71 nmol/L compared with 46 nmol/L).

3. D stimulates production of antimicrobial peptides

Patients with tuberculosis have lower vitamin D levels in blood than control subjects [391-393]. The bacterium that causes TB, Mycobacterium tuberculosis, is an intracellular pathogen that resides predominantly within white blood cells called macrophages. Macrophages possess an enzyme that enables them to change the inactive form of vitamin D3 into the active form. Vitamin D stimulates the production of both antibacterial peptides and lysosomal enzymes in macrophages so enhancing phagocytosis and the cell's defence against mycobacteria [77]. The vitamin also induces the transformation of other white cells called monocytes into macrophages. These activities are important in the defence against TB and other infections and have been well reviewed by Martin Hewison of the University of California School of Medicine [394].

In 1897 Niels Finsen, a Copenhagen doctor, published work describing how tuberculosis of the skin could be cured by directly irradiating it with UV from a carbon-arc lamp which became known as the Finsen lamp. Finsen obtained the Nobel Prize for this work in 1903 and later it was shown that tuberculosis of the skin could be cured by treatment with vitamin D itself [329].

Tuberculosis of the lungs was also treated with sunlight in sanitoria built for the purpose, for example in mountain areas where sunlight is more intense. The sanitoria had rooms arranged so that beds could be moved into the sun [395, 396]. A number of hospitals in the UK, such as Harefield Hospital near London, were also designed in this way. Regrettably, the importance of sunlight for prevention of tuberculosis was forgotten until recently.

Vitamin D levels in old people are generally very low, as a result their immunity declines and this makes them vulnerable to all sorts of infections including shingles. Shingles occurs as a result of the reactivation of infection with the varicella-zoster virus that causes chickenpox [397, 398].

Summary: Low levels of vitamin D in the population are probably an important risk factor for influenza epidemics and other winter virus epidemics that cause severe colds, flu-like illness, bronchitis and pneumonia. These diseases cause a high mortality in old people as well as serious illness and discomfort in people of all ages. They also cost a great deal in lost days from work. Present public health policy is to provide vaccination against flu for old people but questions have been raised about its efficacy. Much winter illness might be prevented if vitamin D supplements were widely taken by the public. Winter circulation of viruses and epidemics of influenza might be much reduced if government recommended and promoted use of vitamin D supplements. Trials are urgently needed.

Chapter 6:
Epidemics on the north Atlantic Islands

The highest incidence of multiple sclerosis in the world was once thought to occur in the Orkney Islands, and in the neighbouring Faroe Islands an "epidemic" of multiple sclerosis is said to have occurred following World War II. About the same time a second "epidemic", this time of leukaemia, occurred among children in Orkney and Shetland. Intensive studies have centred on the theory that these epidemics were caused by infection brought to the islands from outside.

However, evidence that we now have suggests that infectious disease is not a cause of multiple sclerosis (see Chapter 3 above) and intensive research has failed to find an infectious agent that causes leukaemia. Viruses may play a part in multiple sclerosis, but they do not appear to be necessary for it to occur, or if they are involved they are so universally present that they are not a limiting factor. On the other hand much evidence points to insufficient sunlight and/or vitamin D being the major cause, indeed the *sine qua non*, of multiple sclerosis.

In fact the "epidemics" in the north Atlantic islands and differences in incidence of chronic disease may be best understood as part of an historical and geographical narrative: a story of survival in an extreme climate, of fishing, farming and changes in everyday diet brought about by long term economic trends, war and the decline in fish stocks. The reduction in vitamin D in the diet of north Atlantic islanders following historical changes in fishing has increased their vulnerability to diseases caused by vitamin D insufficiency, in particular multiple sclerosis and possibly also childhood leukaemia.

1. Wartime "epidemics" of multiple sclerosis

Between 1943 and 1949 some 20 people in the Faroe Islands developed symptoms of multiple sclerosis in what has been dubbed an epidemic by John F Kurtzke of Georgetown University Medical School, Washington DC. Kurtzke believes that the islanders who developed MS were exposed to an infection brought to the islands by British troops between 1941 and 1944 [399].

The Faroe islands, located at latitude 62° N about halfway between Shetland and Iceland, were in a crucial strategic position in both world wars. British troops occupied the islands, which came under Danish protection, when Denmark itself was threatened and occupied by Hitler's forces. Occupying British troops reached a peak of 7,000 in 1942 declining to about 1,000 or so in 1944.

Kurtzke's research shows that troop encampments were generally located close to the houses of MS patients. He concludes: "The British troops therefore brought something to the Faroese which later resulted in an epidemic of clinical MS. This had to be an infection or a toxin with either one geographically widespread on the islands from 1941." [399]

A further four "epidemics" involving 34 people occurred in the Faroes between 1953 and 1990, according to Kurtzke, but none of these later epidemics were as large as the first post war epidemic [399]. The people who developed MS came as before from villages where British soldiers were encamped during the war. Kurtzke takes this as evidence that the disease was an infection, rather than a toxin, and was transmitted continuously.

Kurtzke believes that the first ever case of multiple sclerosis to occur in the Faroe Islands was diagnosed during World War II in 1943 [399]. Multiple sclerosis could not be found in the island before that date.

More epidemics but are they genuine?

Epidemics of MS also occurred in Orkney, Shetland and Iceland following World War II, according to Kurtzke, providing further evidence for his infection theory [400-402]. In Iceland (63° to 65° N latitude) the incidence of MS appeared to double in 1945 and remained high for 10 years before returning close to its pre-war level [403]. However records show that MS existed in Iceland before World War II; and the increase in numbers of patients diagnosed with the disease in Iceland immediately before, during and after the war coincides with the arrival of two neurologists on the island and completion of a survey that they conducted [404].

Indeed, multiple sclerosis may have occurred in Iceland some 800 years ago during the time of the sagas. Trygve Holmoy, a Norwegian neurologist, has pointed to the Saga of Bishop Thoriak which describes a woman named Halldora, who suffered from transient paralysis between 1193 and 1198 [146]. Nowadays Iceland has an incidence of MS that has settled down to a level between 3.5 and 4.1/100,000 for the post-war period up to the 1990s [404].

This is a relatively low incidence, similar to that for the Mediterranean island of Malta [150].

There are also serious doubts about Kurtzke's claim that an epidemic of multiple sclerosis occurred on the Faroes during and after the war – the increase in cases at that time may just be a random variation of no statistical significance [405, 406]. Kurtzke supposes that people in the Faroe Islands are isolated because the islands are so remote, making them vulnerable to infection brought in from outside. However, the Faroese people have always had many contacts with people in Iceland, Denmark and Shetland. At any one time some 25% of the Faroese are resident abroad. Multiple sclerosis is relatively common in Denmark and other parts of Scandinavia, so if a virus caused the disease the Faroese are likely to have been exposed to it before World War II.

Nevertheless in 1962 a study of multiple sclerosis in Orkney and Shetland found that the disease was some three times more prevalent than anywhere else in the world (309 cases per 100,000 people in Orkney and 184/100,000 in Shetland) [407]. Further studies established that the islands had a high incidence of multiple sclerosis: 7.5 new cases per 100,000 people per year in Shetland and 9.3/100,000 in Orkney between 1940 and 1969 [136]. But a decrease in incidence of the disease occurred on both islands between 1969 and 1986 [401]. Kurtzke took this as a sign that there had been a post war epidemic of MS in Orkney and Shetland [402]. However studies of death certificates suggest that a relatively high incidence of the disease occurred in both island groups from about 1880, and certainly from 1908 when the diagnosis of "disseminated sclerosis" first began to be used [136].

2. An epidemic of leukaemia – Troops blamed again

An epidemic of leukaemia in Orkney and Shetland has also been blamed on the stationing of British troops in the north Atlantic islands during World War Two. The incidence of leukaemia in children increased 3.6 fold in the islands at that time and it has been suggested that forces coming to defend the islands against Hitler brought a novel infection into the community [408]. This is the so-called "population mixing hypothesis". However, no specific infectious agent has been identified as being responsible or even associated with this epidemic of leukaemia.

Mixing of populations elsewhere has also been followed by an increase in childhood leukaemia, for example, around the Dounreay nuclear site and other places where large numbers of incomers mix with a rural population [409, 410]. Infection has been postulated as the most likely cause of these outbreaks but concrete evidence is lacking. Ionising radiation and certain chemicals such as benzene are other suggested causes of leukaemia but there is no special reason to believe that Orkney or Shetland islanders have had any abnormal exposure to these.

Simultaneous epidemics of MS and leukaemia

The reality of the epidemic of multiple sclerosis on the Faroes has been seriously questioned, but if it did occur it was more or less simultaneous with increases in the number of people suffering from multiple sclerosis in Orkney and Shetland and with an epidemic of leukaemia on those islands. These events appear to be linked in time and space. Could they perhaps have a common cause?

Leukaemia is the most common childhood cancer and some 85% of leukaemia cases are of the type known as acute lymphoblastic leukaemia. About 500 cases of childhood leukaemia are diagnosed each year in the UK. About 100 of these children die while the rest have to suffer difficult, demanding and expensive treatment. Leukaemia kills more children each year than any other disease in the UK. So, if the epidemic on Orkney and Shetland can provide any clues, or even just suggest new ideas about the cause of leukaemia this will be worthwhile

Since at least the 1980s it has been known that the active hormone form of vitamin D, calcitriol (1,25 dihydroxycholecalciferol), induces differentiation of human myeloid leukaemic cells and inhibits leukaemic cell proliferation in the test tube [411, 412]. Trials are now under way to find out if these observations can be translated into therapy [413-415].

This should be enough to make vitamin D insufficiency an obvious candidate to explain the leukaemia epidemic in Orkney and Shetland. But infection and radiation have for many years been the fashionable hypotheses that are always considered as the cause of leukaemia. Vitamin D insufficiency is an additional hypothesis that should be considered because of the profound effect of vitamin D on leukaemia cells in the test tube, but somehow it has been overlooked.

At first it seems unlikely that two diseases as different as multiple sclerosis and leukaemia could have much in common, but both diseases are or may be associated with insufficient vitamin D. Reduction in intake of fish, and hence of vitamin D, during World War II is a possible cause of the epidemic of childhood leukaemia in Orkney and Shetland and the apparent increases in multiple sclerosis in these and other north Atlantic islands.

There are other surprising links between these two diseases. Children with leukaemia are up to four times more likely than other children to have a mother who suffers from multiple sclerosis, according to two studies [416, 417]. Babies of women with multiple sclerosis are likely to be at risk of vitamin D insufficiency (see Chapter 3). If leukaemia is caused at least in part by vitamin D insufficiency during pregnancy this could explain why children with leukaemia have a mother with MS more often than might be expected.

3. Prescription – Fish twice a day with meals

The British Isles are an extreme climate providing barely enough sun for healthy living. The islands further north, Orkney, Shetland, Faroes and Iceland, are at an even greater extreme. Orkney (latitude: 59°) and Shetland (latitude: 60°) are the most northerly part of Scotland, while the Faroes, now an independent territory under Danish protection, lie even further north at latitude 62° N, 170 miles north west of Shetland.

The sky above the north Atlantic islands is frequently cloudy or overcast and sunny days are relatively rare. The Faroes have more than 260 rainy days a year, while Shetland has rain on 200 days a year. Shetland gets less UVB in the effective range than Kiruna which is above the Arctic Circle in the very northernmost part of Sweden [23]. Temperatures in summer average only 9 to 12°C so islanders seldom remove clothes and expose much skin to the sun. This means that they get substantially less vitamin D from the sun than people living in southern Scotland. In the past, when islanders ate more fish, this was less of a problem than it is today.

Marine produce of all kinds is a major source of vitamin D for people who live in northern latitudes where the sun is weaker, the summer is shorter and the climate colder. A 100 gm portion of fish can provide between 400 and 1600 IUs of vitamin D [418]. Small fish eaten with their bones are also a good source of calcium, which has a sparing action on utilisation of vitamin D. Two fish meals per day, whether the fish is fresh, dried or smoked, could provide up to 2000 IUs of vitamin D. If this were kept up year round it would provide enough vitamin D for good health, indeed probably better health than that of most Scots today.

The way in which increased fish in the diet can compensate for less sun exposure is shown by observations from Norway. People living in southern Norway (Vest-Agder, latitude: 58°) get about 50% more exposure to UV light than those living in the north (Finnmark, latitude: 70°) and so the southerners synthesise correspondingly more vitamin D. But the inhabitants of Finnmark eat about 25% more fish than the southern Norwegians. The result is that Norwegians from both ends of the country end up with closely similar average levels of vitamin D [419].

It may not be possible for inhabitants of the north Atlantic islands to remain healthy and reach a good old age unless they eat fish regularly or, nowadays, take a vitamin D supplement. It is in this context that the changes in incidence of multiple sclerosis and leukaemia on the islands may be explained. Several, apparently conflicting, questions need to be answered:

1) Could there be a link between apparent increases in multiple sclerosis in the islands and the epidemic of leukaemia that occurred on Orkney and Shetland at about the same time?

2) Is it possible to explain why multiple sclerosis occurred for many years before World War II in Iceland, Orkney and Shetland but not apparently in the Faroes?

3) The incidence of multiple sclerosis in Iceland is relatively low whereas the incidence in Orkney and Shetland reached world record levels for a period. How can that be explained?

4) Why has Scotland got the highest incidence of multiple sclerosis in the world? – details in Chapter 3.

A diet of seabirds, fish and pilot whale

The north Atlantic islanders, like other seafaring people round the Scottish coast, had found a successful way of living in a difficult environment in the pre-industrial age. The original diet of the indigenous Norse and Scottish islanders was probably similar to that of inhabitants of the island of St Kilda 100 years ago [420]. The diet of the people on this isolated island 40 miles west of Uist in the Hebrides was recorded before the island was evacuated in 1930. They ate seabirds such as Fulmar, gannet and puffin, and birds' eggs obtained by scaling the cliffs on long ropes, as well as all types of fish. Their diet contained few if any fresh vegetables. The traditional diet of the Faroes, which was still eaten well into the 20th century and continues for some today, is similar: fresh or dried fish, puffins and their eggs, dried mutton, blubber and meat from the pilot whale.

This diet seems very strange to us nowadays, but it was ideally suited to their relatively sunless climate. Today the north Atlantic islands have become modernised. The North Sea oil industry has changed Shetland and undersea tunnels or bridges now connect many of the Faroe Islands. Orkney has a flourishing farm business. So while some may still eat the traditional diet others can now buy a modern convenience diet, including hamburger and fries at the Burger King restaurant in Torshavn, capital of the Faroe Islands.

Traditionally fishermen in the Scottish islands went out in open boats called sixareens rowed by six men, and in small sailing smacks [421]. A trade in dried and salted fish had existed in the northern islands for more than three hundred years. But the traditional life style of Scotland's fishermen began to change fundamentally at the end of the 19th and beginning of the 20th centuries.

In the second half of the 19th century fish stocks in the North Sea became badly depleted by the large fleets of sailing boats that had increased in size as the market for fresh fish expanded. The development of fish markets and railways on mainland Britain enabled rapid sale and distribution of catches. But change became even more rapid at the turn of the 19th century with the development of steam trawlers that enabled much greater catches to be taken. These boats could go further afield to find the fish and take them back for sale in mainland markets such as Aberdeen*.

Deep-sea fishermen employed on these trawlers would be away for a week or more at a time. When they returned they received wages that became more important for their families than the fish they caught. Also fish itself became more expensive as local stocks were depleted and trawlers had to go further away to the waters around Iceland and Bear Island (Svalbard). And so families began to buy the usual industrial food items of 19th and 20th century Britain: flour, sugar and saturated fat, or bread and other baked goods such as scones, shortbread and tea-breads which consist mainly of white flour and sugar with variable amounts of fat. As they ate less fish, and other marine food items such as seabirds, the vitamin D levels of Scots fishing communities must have declined.

The herring fishery, which began each year round Shetland, was transformed by the use of steam powered boats. At the end of the 19th century only a small percentage of herring drifters had steam power but by the start of the First World War about 80% of the English and Welsh fleet were powered by steam and similar changes occurred in Scotland.

Trawlers hunted by submarines

During the First World War trawlers were pressed into service to hunt submarines and clear mines while the fishermen's experience of the sea made them invaluable in the Navy. In 1916 alone 156 steam trawlers were sunk by enemy action in the North Sea. The fish stocks began to recover, but the men serving in the navy became accustomed to a different type of food. At home fish was not so readily available during the war because fishing was dangerous, and women had wages from the men serving in the forces to spend on other types of food.

By the time the First World War ended fish stocks had recovered and there were great catches in the North Sea for a few years but at home the daily diet had already begun to change. Technical developments enabled fishing to continue to be profitable, at least in the short term. Large scale production of ice enabled catches to be preserved longer before reaching the market, helping the deep-sea trawlers that voyaged to Iceland and the Polar seas north of Norway. But by the 1930s the bonanza in the North Sea had ended and fishermen once again were having a hard time finding catches. The UK government became convinced that something needed to be done and in 1933 new laws were brought in to regulate mesh sizes of nets and landing sizes of the main species of fish.

The scarcity of fish in the 1930s accelerated changes that were already occurring in the diet of islanders. The Department of Health for Scotland reporting on Scotland as a whole noted in 1936 that witnesses "deplored the passing of the old staple foods of porridge, salt herring and potatoes and the substitution of shop bread, tinned foods, tea and sweets and other goods purchased from shops or more commonly traders' vans". [422]

Even so some Scots doctors thought that the diet was improving with increased consumption of butchers' meat and the introduction of fruits such as apples, oranges and bananas. But others remarked: "Tinned corned beef is constantly asked for. Pastries and cheap sweets are extensively sold by the vans ... As far as I can gather the Highland child is drinking 60 per cent less fresh milk than it did in the pre-war [pre 1914-18] period ... Seldom now does the crofter fish." [422]

These changes in diet were occurring in all but the most remote parts of the Scottish Islands. An inquiry undertaken by the Medical Research Council into the diet of families in the Highlands and Islands of Scotland in the late 1930s found that people on the island of Lewis still ate fish regularly [423]. The average Lewis family ate 13.5 lbs of fish per week, more than half of it fatty fish. This is about half a pound of fish a day for each family member providing about 1500 IUs of vitamin D, an amount sufficient for basic good health. In the more remote south

---

• I first learnt about the fishing industry as a child in North Shields during regular visits to the Fish Quay with my father. Trawlers from the Scottish east coast could always be seen in the harbour. In the late 1940s or early 1950s the occasional converted sailing boat with its mast cut off and a diesel engine could still be seen. In the later 1950s and 1960s larger stern trawlers that could haul their catch up a ramp at the back of the boat began to appear. However I am much indebted here to Professor Callum Roberts' book: *The unnatural history of the sea: The past and future of humanity and fishing.* (Gaia publishing, London, 2007)

eastern coastal districts of the island families ate even more fish, particularly herring [345].

Traditional fish dishes eaten on Lewis included boiled cod's head and stomach of cod stuffed with chopped cod's liver, onions and oatmeal. Crude cod liver oil was used traditionally in the more remote areas as a food. But J.D.King, a dentist surveying the islanders teeth, remarks that these once popular items had become rare on the Lewis-man's menu by the late 1930s [345]. He also notes that a better ferry service with the mainland, improvement in the island's roads, the arrival of the Scottish Co-operative Wholesale Society shops on the island, and the distribution of food through tradesmen's vans, were responsible for changes in the islanders' diet. Similar changes were occurring all over Scotland including Shetland [421].

4. Wartime rationing – one egg every two months

In 1939 the outbreak of war forced many more people to change to a modern industrial diet, albeit of the most basic kind. Military restrictions and minefields placed the North Sea off-limits, allowing only inshore fishing. Thousands of soldiers and navy personnel were stationed on Orkney and Shetland to defend it against hostile action and to exercise control over the North Sea. And when Denmark fell to the Nazis, Allied forces also occupied the Faroe Islands to prevent Hitler obtaining a convenient base for his submarines.

Some 60,000 servicemen were stationed on Orkney and Shetland during World War II and some 40,000 sailors remained at the ready on boats sheltering in Scapa Flow, the large natural harbour in Orkney. In addition, in Orkney, there were some 3,700 construction workers, 1,200 Italian prisoners and 2,000 refugees from Norway. These incomers outnumbered the local population of the two islands, which was just over 40,000 [408].

The service personnel, prisoners and others were all fed in the usual way by large-scale supplies of potatoes, flour, sugar and animal fat imported from the mainland. Food was of course rationed and so it would certainly be supplemented with fish when this was possible but large supplies of fish were difficult or impossible to get during the war because of the risk to boats.

During World War II rationing severely restricted eggs and meat, which were the only foods, other than fish, that contained any vitamin D. In 1941, for example, eggs were limited to one per person every two months. Meat was available only in very small quantities and continued to be rationed throughout the UK until 1954. The men folk serving in the navy learned of necessity to eat the wartime rations. So the trend towards a modern industrial diet similar to that eaten by most other people in the UK continued, even though it was low in vitamin D and not suited to people living so far north.

The war once more saved fish stocks. When it ended in 1945 there was another brief glut of good catches before stocks were again reduced to levels that made fishing in home waters marginal. Fishermen who could afford it invested in larger more powerful boats with stern ramps for hauling in the trawl and freezers that could preserve the fish immediately they were caught. But these large catches mostly went for sale on the mainland. Fisher folk continued to eat more meat, bread and other familiar foods found in the shops.

Meat eaten instead of fish

By 1967 consumption of fish by rural people on the island of Lewis (Hebrides) had halved and the diet of urban people living in the major town on the island, Stornaway, was noted to be very similar to other parts of the UK with children commonly eating fish in the form of ready prepared fish fingers. The most significant change in the diet was a substitution of meat for fish resulting in a decline in vitamin D consumption together with a decline in the consumption of calcium. A survey of children's teeth on the island showed a notable decline in their dental health since the previous survey some 30 years earlier – see Chapter 4 [424]. These changes, so well documented in the Island of Lewis, occurred all over Scotland as modern industrial patterns of living and our modern industrial diet arrived in previously remote regions. Similar changes occurred in Shetland as recorded by Cluness [421].

It is easy to see that during a period of 100 or more years there was a varying but remorseless pressure to move away from the traditional marine diet in the north Atlantic islands. Going back 200 years they would probably have eaten fish twice a day. But after two World Wars and two major crises in the supply of fish islanders became dependent on wages to obtain food. Changes in incidence of disease and occurrence of epidemics on the different islands may be accounted for by the way in which their diet was influenced at various times by war, availability of wage earning jobs and penetration of the local economy by retailers.

A survey of lifetime events in MS patients on Orkney and Shetland has endeavoured to find an exposure to some infectious agent or environmental insult that could be the cause of the disease. More of the MS patients lived in the small island towns, in Kirkwall and Stromness on Orkney and in Lerwick on Shetland, than in the more remote rural areas, but otherwise their lives and habits were remarkably similar to those of the controls. Shetland patients seemed to enjoy potted head (made from pig's head) more often than controls and some were less exposed to animals but the differences were not large enough to provide significant leads [425]. Other aspects of diet were not investigated and so it is not known if there were any differences in consumption of fish between MS patients and others.

The sea provides a relatively complete diet. But the modern industrial diet that has replaced it lacks not only vitamin D, it may also lack fresh vegetables, especially in Scotland where, because of the limitations of climate, vegetables have always been less favoured than in England [426].* In common with other cancers, leukaemia and malignancies of blood cells (haemopoeitic malignancies) occur less frequently in people who have a diet with plenty of vegetables and fruits [428].

Other studies have shown that a high body mass index and obesity are associated with an increased risk of leukaemia as well as other cancers [429]. The dietary changes that occurred in the north Atlantic Islands as a result of declining fish stocks and wartime rationing favoured starchy diets and, if continued when food became more plentiful, would tend to cause increased body weight. As the World Cancer Research Fund report, edited by Sir Michael Marmot, makes clear: "Obesity results in pathological states of inflammation and altered immune responses, both of which are factors that can influence ... haemopoietic cell function."

And so the change in diet in the north Atlantic islands, most evident during World War II, may have put people at risk of leukaemia by the synergistic decrease in vitamin D intake together with an increase in intake of calories with few vegetables. The interaction of these two factors may explain changes in incidence of leukaemia both geographically and over time.

5. Two diseases with something in common

The temporary increase in incidence of leukaemia in Orkney and Shetland contrasts with a steady increase in incidence in the rest of the UK and in Nordic countries. Leukaemia has become more common in children in the UK over the last 50 years or more, as have other diseases that appear to be caused in part by D insufficiency: diabetes type 1, multiple sclerosis and Crohn's disease – see chapter 3 [430, 431].

Lymphoblastic leukaemia has increased in North West England at an average rate of 0.7% per year during the last 50 years of the 20th century and in Sweden at a similar rate of 0.85% per year [432]. Incidence of leukaemia in British girls increased by 57% between 1979 and 1990 with a similar increase in the Nordic countries [433].

The parallel increase in these diseases suggests a change in what might be a common environmental factor. That factor seems likely to be vitamin D insufficiency since it is a known risk factor for two of the four diseases. A further link between diabetes type 1 and multiple sclerosis supports the suggestion that they have a common cause.

People with multiple sclerosis and their relatives have been found to suffer more frequently than would be expected from diabetes type 1 and *vice versa* [434-436]. While genetics is likely to be involved, the rapid increase in incidence of these diseases over the years suggests that there is a common environmental trigger, almost certainly vitamin D insufficiency.

A correlation has also been found between the incidence of acute lymphoblastic leukaemia and the incidence of diabetes type 1, both in Europe and in other parts of the world where statistics are available [430]. Again this suggests these two diseases may have a common cause. Finally, deaths from leukaemia at all ages are greatest in those parts of the United States that get least UV-B from sunlight, supporting the suggestion that sunlight may be a factor in the disease [437].

---

* Potatoes and vegetables other than perhaps peas and kail (a coarse variety of cabbage) did not become a common part of the Highland and Island diet until the middle of the 18th century. Before that time the Scots diet consisted mainly of oatmeal, barley (knock-it bere), dairy produce (milk, butter and crowdie), fish and occasional beef or mutton. In 1808 Dr John Walker recorded: "At no very remote period, the common productions of the kitchen garden were unknown in the Highlands [or islands]. Lochiel, on returning from abroad with excellent intentions to improve his country, established a kitchen garden at his seat at Achnacary; and in August 1734 entertained his guests with hotch-potch containing pease, turnips and carrots which was the first time these vegetables had been produced in that part of the world. Since that time kitchen gardens have been formed at all the gentlemen's houses: but the common tenants and subtenants remain still destitute of a garden of any kind." [427]. Walker, J., *An Economic History of the Hebrides and Highlands of Scotland*. 1808, London. By the 19th century potatoes had become a staple part of the diet of the north Atlantic islanders and like the Irish, they suffered terribly during the potato famines in the middle of the century [421] Cluness, A., *The Shetland Isles*. 1951, London: Hale.

6. Leukaemia – an event in pregnancy

Leukaemia in childhood appears to arise from an event during pregnancy which causes chromosome breaks with improper repair [438, 439]. It has been suggested that the event may be infection followed by a failure of immune system modulation [440]. However, modulation of the immune system can fail as a result of insufficient vitamin D in the absence of any infection. (For a description of vitamin D modulation of the immune system see Chapter 3.) So it seems equally reasonable to suggest that the crucial event leading to childhood leukaemia might be vitamin D insufficiency followed by failure of normal differentiation of immune cells during early life.

Some 70% of children with leukaemia have been found to have abnormally low plasma 1,25-dihydroxyvitamin D levels at diagnosis [441]. This could be a consequence of the disease itself but is also consistent with the causal process suggested here.

The events leading to childhood leukaemia caused by vitamin D insufficiency might then be seen as follows. White blood cells fail to differentiate normally because vitamin D levels are insufficient. These abnormal cells persist longer than usual in the bone marrow and as they age chromosome breaks occur by chance. Generally such aberrant cells, with or without chromosome breaks, would be destroyed by apoptosis (programmed death of cells), but in absence of sufficient vitamin D apoptosis does not occur. So these cells persist in the marrow for an unusually long time. At any rate, time enough for selection of cell lines that are immortal. These immortal cell lines, or cancer clones, are able to multiply without restriction leading to a peak in the first two years of life in the case of acute myeloid leukaemia and in the third or fourth year of life in the case of acute lymphocytic leukaemia.

Leukaemia birthdays more likely in spring or summer

Children with leukaemia living in northern climates are more likely to have birthdays in spring or summer, according to scientific evidence reviewed below. As with multiple sclerosis and diabetes type 1, low vitamin D levels during pregnancies ending in spring and early summer may be the cause, although seasonal virus infections could also trigger the disease. I provide summary details of the scientific evidence below so that readers may see that while interesting it is not conclusive.

In one study seasonal trends were looked for in the birthdays of 4,199 children under 15 in northern England who had been diagnosed with all types of cancer. Birthdays of children aged 1 to 6 with acute lymphoblastic leukaemia showed a seasonal trend, but there was no seasonal trend in birthdays of children with other cancers. The children with this type of leukaemia who lived in northern England including Cumbria were more likely to have birthdays in early spring, while those in Yorkshire showed a weaker trend for birthdays bunching in late summer [442].

A study of 961 children in the US who died of leukaemia and 1,552 children who died of cancer when under a year old found that the birthdays of those with leukaemia peaked in May while birthdays of children with other cancers showed no seasonal pattern [443]. A third study of 20,949 children in the United States found a seasonal summer peak of birthdays of children with acute lymphoblastic leukaemia. Seasonal peaks were also found for rhabdomyosarcoma and hepatoblastoma [444].

The fact that a seasonal distribution of birthdays has been more commonly found for leukaemia than for most other cancers in three different studies suggests it may be a real effect. It appears that a seasonal factor acting in spring or summer, probably when vitamin D levels are lowest, has a role in causing acute lymphoblastic leukaemia in young children. It needs to be remembered here that vitamin D levels of people living in northern latitudes are often not replenished until late summer when holidays are most commonly taken.

Further support for a spring or summer date as the time when this seasonal factor is most likely to act comes from a Danish study of 458 children under 4 years old who had acute lymphoblastic leukaemia and whose birthdays bunched in April [445]. And another study of 61 children under 4 who had become known to the charity Children with Leukaemia found that almost half of them (28 out of 61) had their birthdays in March, April or May [446].

Two large studies, one from the US and one from the UK, have failed to confirm a clear seasonal trend in birthdays of children with acute lymphoblastic leukaemia [447, 448]. However, when the data in the US study was subdivided geographically a seasonal peak was found in January in the northern United States although this was not remarked on in the authors' conclusions. And the UK study did find a significant February peak in birthdays of children with leukaemia born before 1960.

7. Cancer and Crohn's in the North Atlantic islands

Other diseases that appear to be caused by insufficient vitamin D were less common than might be expected in the Faroes, Shetland and Orkney during the post-World War II period.

The incidence of rectum and colon cancer in the Faroe islands between 1989 and 1993 was among the lowest in north-western Europe and North America according to scientists at the Institute of Cancer Epidemiology in Copenhagen [449]. The incidence of rectal cancer during this period was 60% that of Denmark, where the people have a closely similar genetic background, and the incidence of colon cancer was 75% of that in Denmark.

Of all cancers those of the bowel, including the colon and rectum, appear to be most sensitive to the level of vitamin D in the body [450-453]. This finding is consistent with that of the Physicians' Health Study, which found the risk of colorectal cancer was reduced by 40% over a 22 year period in those men who ate most fish [454]. Vitamin D content of the diet was not measured because the investigators' hypothesis was that long chain n-3 fatty acids (Omega-3) in fish are protective against colorectal cancer.

The incidence of Crohn's disease on the Faroe Islands is low, 1.75 cases per 100,000 people, compared with other countries [455]. In Iceland the incidence is higher at 4.5 per 100,000 [243]. While in Shetland the incidence is 5.7 per 100,000 and in Orkney 6.1 per 100,000. In northeastern Scotland the incidence of Crohn's disease was 9.8 per 100,000, "the highest recorded from a mixed urban and rural community"[243]. While in Aberdeen the incidence reached 11.6 per 100,000 during the three years 1985-87. All these figures of incidence come from surveys completed in the 1980s.

As discussed above, Crohn's seems to be caused at least in part by low levels of vitamin D. It seems likely that the differences in incidence of Crohn's disease between these northern locations may be explained by the amount of fish and hence vitamin D in the diet.

The Danish epidemiologists comment in their article on cancer in the Faroes: "This relatively low risk of colorectal cancer occurs in spite of a low intake of vegetables and a high intake of total fat. However the Faroese diet is high in fish, calcium and vitamin D and the possibility therefore exists that the low rates are due to a protective effect of these nutrients and micronutrients."

Recommendations for prevention of cancer based on epidemiology have emphasised consumption of vegetables [428]. However a high fish or high vitamin D diet may be another effective way of reducing risk of some cancers even when vegetable intake is low.

Summary: The epidemic of leukaemia in Orkney and Shetland, the apparent epidemic of multiple sclerosis in the Faroes, and differences in incidence of multiple sclerosis in the north Atlantic islands and in other parts of Scotland, together with the low incidence of colorectal cancer and Crohn's disease in the Faroes, may be explained, at least in part, by historical changes in availability of fish during the last century. A study identifying the epidemic of leukaemia in Orkney and Shetland did not consider that the outbreak of the disease in these islands may have been caused by insufficient vitamin D. It is surprising that this explanation has been overlooked because it has biological plausibility and is consistent with other findings. Future research needs to consider vitamin D insufficiency as a contributor to risk of childhood leukaemia.

Chapter 7:
A new Public Health Policy for sunlight and vitamin D

1. Full review not undertaken by government advisors

In May 2007 the UK's Scientific Advisory Committee on Nutrition (SACN) published a report *Update on Vitamin D* that has been followed by some significant but limited changes in UK government policy on vitamin D. The SACN report stated: "New data continue to emerge regarding the health benefits of vitamin D. Although a full systematic review was not undertaken, much evidence suggests that vitamin D may be implicated in a wide range of other diseases including osteoporosis, several forms of cancer, cardiovascular disease, tuberculosis, multiple sclerosis and type 1 diabetes. Both osteoporosis and osteomalacia increase the risk of fractures."

While SACN clearly acknowledges much evidence for the health benefits of vitamin D, it omitted, as it says itself, to undertake a full review. As a result of this omission SACN was unable to appreciate the full force of scientific evidence that is available. Even so SACN did not hesitate to say that the evidence was inconclusive and to call for more definitive evidence.

As a result the English Department of Health in London, which has acted for the UK as a whole in this matter, has taken no action to recommend any increase in vitamin D levels of adults in the UK. The official view remains that adults in the UK who are mobile and able to go out of the home obtain sufficient vitamin D by casual exposure to the sun. This is quite extraordinary when the low levels of vitamin D in the UK have been so comprehensively documented by Hypponen and others [5, 456].

Nevertheless there has been an important change in UK health policy on sun exposure that was marked in December 2007 by a limited promotion of vitamin D to pregnant and nursing mothers. The new advice from government clearly recognises that food alone does not provide enough vitamin D – at least for mothers – and this is an important step forward. The risk of rickets is also emphasised in this new advice that warns: "Healthcare professionals are concerned at the increasing numbers of children at risk of vitamin D deficiency in the UK".

2. UK government now recommends sunshine – and bare shoulders

"It takes only 15 minutes exposure of the arms, head and shoulders in the sun each day during the summer months to make enough vitamin D for good health," the UK Department of Health now advises. "Eating foods like oily fish, eggs, fortified cereals and breads are all sources of vitamin D, but these may still be inadequate when sunshine hours are limited. At these times pregnant and breastfeeding women and children under four may benefit from a supplement containing 10 micrograms [400 IUs] of vitamin D."

A 15 minutes per day exposure to the sun is a major advance on previous official advice recommending that casual exposure of the hands and face is sufficient. The logic of the previous advice was quite simple: what you get is all you need. In fact there was never any scientific evidence to support the suggestion that such limited exposure is sufficient [457]. So the new advice suggesting that 15 minutes exposure per day of arms, head and shoulders to the sun is a major step forward – particularly the recommendation of bare shoulders which have never been mentioned before.

Longer sun exposures needed for optimum D

The new government advice is directed at pregnant women, but if the advice is considered safe for pregnant women then it ought also to be safe for other adults. The new advice appears to be based on the SACN report which takes as its authority on sun exposure a journal article by Dr Michael Holick [29] and this in turn refers to Dr Holick's book *The UV Advantage* published in 2003, in which he describes the "Holick formula for safe sun" [458]. It is clear from Holick's book that the government's recommendation of a 15 minute per day exposure of face, arms, and shoulders is in fact a minimum recommended time. Inspection of Holick's "Safe Sun Tables" [458] shows that a 15 minute exposure has been calculated by Holick to provide a light skinned person in the UK with between 800 and 1,500 IUs of vitamin D. If shoulders are bared as well then vitamin D synthesis will certainly be nearer the higher figure.

However. the 15-minute exposure must be made at around midday in high summer (June, July or August) if it is to provide the calculated amount of vitamin D. According to Holick's tables a person sunning themselves outside the midday period (i.e. outside the hours 12pm to 3pm) will have to remain in the sun two or three times longer to get the same benefit – or remove more clothes. And outside the high summer period, in April, May and September, the sun is much less strong in midday than it is in midsummer. So in these early or late months of summer it is necessary to stay in the sun much longer than 15 minutes or expose more flesh to obtain the suggested dose of vitamin D.

Furthermore Holick's calculations were made when it was thought that 1000 IUs of vitamin D per day were more than enough. It is now thought that more like 4,000 IUs per day are needed. When all these considerations are taken together Holick's figure of 15 minutes sun exposure per day must be multiplied by about 10 for optimum generation of vitamin D and optimum health. Obviously a 150 minute (10 x 15 minutes) exposure to the sun is too long. So, instead of exposing only hands, face and shoulders, the whole body should be exposed for a shorter time to increase the area of skin working to produce vitamin D while avoiding burning.

There are additional reasons to increase sun exposure over and above the 15 minutes per day to hands, face and shoulders recommended by the government. The most important for readers of this book is that neither Holick nor the UK Health Department makes any allowance for the difference in strength of the sun between England and Scotland. In fact Scots must on average spend some 30-50% longer in the sun, or expose correspondingly more flesh, to get the same benefit as southern English people.

Furthermore a person with darker skin takes up to six or ten times as long to make the same amount of vitamin D as a white person because the dark skin pigment filters out the active UVB rays. So a dark skinned person will need to expose much more than just the hands, arms and face to get the same dose as a light skinned person gets on these areas of skin in 15 minutes. A darker person may need to double or triple their exposure time, which should not be a problem for darker skin provided the subject begins cautiously with short exposures.

Bare as much of the body as possible

When all these considerations are put together it becomes clear that a 15 minute exposure, while useful, is not going to supply optimum vitamin D [459]. It helps if the shoulders are bared as well as arms and face, but it is not sufficient. In any case British men don't generally wear sleeveless vests that bare their shoulders except on very casual occasions, and in Scotland it will mostly be too cold in summer for either men or women to bare their shoulders casually.

So full advantage must be taken of warm sun when it occurs. It makes sense to bare as much of the body as possible and to sunbathe whenever the weather is warm enough and it is convenient and appropriate to remove clothes. Vitamin D generated on good sunny days is then stored and can be used by the body on other days and in winter when the sun is not strong enough to make any vitamin D. So sunbathing makes sense provided care is taken to avoid burning.

The UK Health Protection Agency has precise data on the amount of UVB reaching earth at some five ground stations that it manages at different latitudes across the UK, including ground stations at Glasgow, Kinloss and Lerwick. In 2006 I asked the Agency to use this data to calculate the length of exposure needed for a person to obtain optimum vitamin D at various UK locations at various times of day and times of year. If this were done better guidance could be given to the public on the length of sun exposure needed to get sufficient vitamin D.

Even the Australian authorities are now questioning their passionately promoted advice to avoid the sun and their slip, slap, slop routine* which has provided Cancer Research UK with a model for its SunSmart programme [460]. This follows the discovery that vitamin D insufficiency and even deficiency is quite common in Australia because extreme advice has reinforced the modern trend to live indoors and avoid direct sunlight. Furthermore multiple sclerosis has been found to be several times more common among Australians living in temperate Tasmania than it is among Australians living in sub-tropical Queensland. In a remarkable *volte face* a syndicate of Australian health organisations** recommended in 2005 that Australians get some regular sun exposure each week, especially in the south of the country in winter, before covering up with clothes and sunblock [461, 462].

For years children in Australia have been made to wear hats during outdoor playtime regardless of season or latitude. "No hat. No play", has been the teachers' guiding phrase throughout the continent. Now Tasmanians in the far south of the country, where there is comparatively little sun in winter, have rebelled. Dr Roscoe Taylor,

---

* slip on a shirt, slap on a hat and slop on suncream.
** a position statement on the risks and benefits of sun exposure was approved in 2005 by the Australian and New Zealand Bone and Mineral Society, Osteoporosis Australia, the Australasian College of Dermatologists and The Cancer Council of Australia.

Tasmania's director of public health, has formulated a new "hats off" policy in winter. He urged Tasmanian children to take off their hats and soak up the sun during the winter months. He said people should not compromise their vitamin D levels and be SunSmart when it was not necessary.

3. Risks and benefits of sun exposure: 2,000:1 in favour of exposure

For a clear analysis of the risks and benefits of sun exposure we must look once more to Australia. It is ironic that thinking on the risks and benefits of sun exposure has forged ahead in Australia, while the UK remains lumbered with outdated advice originally devised in Australia for limiting the dangers of the sub-tropical sun.

Dr Robyn Lucas at the Australian National University in Canberra and colleagues have calculated the risk to health and life from sun exposure or the lack of it [463]. In effect they have calculated what might be expected to happen if everybody in the UK obeyed implicitly the original advice of Cancer Research UK (CR-UK) and the UK government, which instructed us to avoid all substantial sun exposure. These official instructions were to put on suncream 20 minutes before going into the sun, to always cover up (CR-UK slogan: "Keep your shirt on"), wear a hat, and to stay in the shade between 11am and 3pm*.

It is not difficult for most people in the UK, whose life is in any case mainly indoors, to follow such instructions to the letter and in so doing avoid sun exposure entirely. Many people in the UK accepted this advice in good faith, did what was advised and as a result obtained no effective sun exposure, obtained virtually no vitamin D other than the very small amount available from food, and put themselves at great risk of serious illness or death.

CR-UK's advice may have saved some lives from skin cancer as they predicted, but for every life saved or disability prevented by such advice some 2,000 lives are expected to have been lost, or equivalent disabilities induced, from bone diseases alone – that is from diseases such as rickets, osteoporosis and fractures [463]. In fact CR-UK's sun avoidance advice must have resulted in even more overall deaths and disability, because deaths and disability from cancer, heart disease, raised blood pressure, stroke, multiple sclerosis and all the other complications of vitamin D insufficiency outlined above are not included in this calculation.

There are some 2,000 deaths from skin cancer a year in the UK. The measures suggested by CR-UK might possibly have saved half of them although this is by no means certain because the major cause of death, melanoma, is not well understood. Burning rather than simple sun exposure appears to be the factor that may increase the risk of melanoma while vitamin D may do something to prevent the disease [464]. Nevertheless the cost of attempting to save a substantial portion, say 1,000, of these 2,000 lives would be two million premature deaths or disability equivalents from bone diseases and an untold number, almost certainly far larger, from cancer and the other diseases mentioned above [109].

Explaining the calculation above in more detail, Dr Lucas and colleagues estimated the global burden of death, disease and disability caused by sun exposure, or lack of it, in units called "disability adjusted life years" or DALYs. This involves identifying diseases such as skin cancer caused by exposure to the sun and using established observations to calculate a population attributable fraction (PAF) - this is the fraction by which the incidence of the disease could be reduced if exposure to the risk factor were eliminated; that is if exposure to the sun is prevented. Disability caused by each disease is also taken into consideration in this calculation and weighted according to intensity and the length of time the disability is endured.

Dr Lucas and colleagues concluded that UV exposure is a minor contributor to the world's disease burden causing an estimated annual burden of 1.6 million DALYs, mostly from skin cancer. This is only 0.1% of the total global disease burden. But they went on to estimate the loss of benefits provided by sun exposure and concluded: "A markedly larger annual disease burden, 3.3 billion DALYs, might result from reduction in global UV exposure to very low levels."

This means that for every one DALY of risk that is prevented by avoiding the sun 2,000 DALYs of benefits of sun are lost if exposure is reduced in the way that was advised by Cancer Research UK and government. These odds are calculated by taking the ratio of 3.3 billion DALYs of disease and death, mostly bone disease, incurred by reducing exposure to the sun versus 1.6 million DALYs of disease and death, mostly from skin cancer, that might be prevented by the same measures.

The reason for this high ratio is explained by Dr Lucas and Dr A.L. Ponsonby in another article [465]. "Although diseases caused by excessive UV exposure are extremely common they tend to occur in older age groups and be relatively benign, thus incurring a relatively low burden of disease despite their high prevalence. In contrast, disorders of UV insufficiency and deficiency affect the young as well as older persons.

---

* CR-UK's advice changed slightly in 2006 - see details of change in their policy in Box 2 page 58.

"Vitamin D deficiency causes infantile rickets, and both rickets and sub-clinical vitamin D deficiency are associated with increased risk of pneumonia and death. Deformities following infantile rickets cause a lasting burden of disease, while osteoporosis and muscle weakness in the elderly contributes to falls and their sequelae, skeletal fractures. The burden of disease avoided by maintaining adequate vitamin D levels or adequate levels of sun exposure, even considering only diseases of the muscloskeletal system, is enormous."

4. Westminster bungles supply of infant vitamins

In December 2007 the UK government advised mothers to take 400 IUs vitamin D daily and to give their babies Healthy Start infant vitamin drops that provide 300 IUs of vitamin D per day. However the Healthy Start infant vitamins, which are a new product manufactured specially according to a government devised formula, are not widely available [93, 466]. The Healthy Start programme is organised centrally from London but the Healthy Start infant vitamins must be ordered and paid for by local Health Trusts and Boards. Many Trusts and Boards have failed to order the infant vitamins and so they are available in only a few areas and are, or have been, unobtainable in Edinburgh, Tayside and many other parts of Scotland.

The original intention was that the Healthy Start infant vitamins would be sold through chemists as infant vitamins were previously when they were known as NHS infant vitamin drops. However in most places Healthy Start infant vitamins appear to be available only to mothers on benefits. This policy makes no sense because occurrence of vitamin D insufficiency is not related to social class or financial status.

It is vital that these vitamins are made available for children in Scotland because evidence suggests that adequate sources of vitamin D in early life can not only provide strong bones but can also prevent rickets, infant heart failure, diabetes type 1 and multiple sclerosis. Multiple sclerosis is a devastating disease that causes increasingly severe handicap and premature death. It has a higher incidence in Scotland than any other country in the world.

Risk for babies born in spring

Scots born in May, after the long, dark winter, have a higher than average risk of MS, while those born in November, after the summer holidays, have the lowest risk [133]. This suggests that a rigorous programme providing vitamin D supplements of the right strength to pregnant mothers and infants could reduce the incidence of multiple sclerosis by 25% or more simply by providing a winter supplement of vitamin D. The risk of rickets, heart failure, and diabetes type 1 would expect to be reduced too. (See earlier sections above for more information about rickets, heart failure in infants, diabetes type 1, and MS).

Vitamin D supplements are important for all women in Scotland because of the climate, but they are especially important for Asian and Afro-Caribbean women during pregnancy in Scotland. The risk of rickets has been found to be much higher in Asian families, particularly if the women are veiled [36, 307, 466]. This is because Asian mothers tend to have low vitamin D levels as a result of their dark skin, which takes longer to make vitamin D than white skin, and their cultural preference for all-enveloping clothes that drastically reduce sun exposure. Osteomalacia is a particular problem in Asian immigrants in the UK. It may emerge in a florid form during pregnancy when the future health of the foetus as well as the mother is at risk [467].

The daily dose of 400 IUs vitamin D recommended for pregnant women by the UK Department of Health as part of the Healthy Start programme is too low. It is not sufficient to sustain circulating levels of vitamin D and does not provide a suitable level of vitamin D in breast milk [468]. Babies that are breast fed, particularly when breast-feeding continues longer than six months, are at high risk of developing rickets and other vitamin D insufficiency diseases.

The Canadian Paediatric Society (CPS) recognizes the special risk for children living in its northern territories that have the same latitude as Scotland. In November 2007 the CPS recommended that pregnant and breast feeding women consult their medical adviser about getting 2,000 IUs vitamin D daily. The CPS also recommended a higher dose of vitamin D for infants: 400 IUs per day in summer and 800 IUs per day in winter for infants living north of latitude 55° north. All of Scotland is above latitude 55° north, except for Wigtownshire and a piece of Kirkcudbrightshire,

A supplement of 2000 IUs vitamin D in pregnancy as recommended by the CPS may be expected to reduce the risks of pre-eclampsia (also known as toxaemia of pregnancy) which is marked by high blood pressure with swelling of hands and feet. Pre-eclampsia is considered to be a major cause of premature delivery, and of deaths of babies and mothers. Bodnar *et al* found that "Low vitamin D early in pregnancy was associated with a five fold increase in odds of pre-eclampsia" [20]. Provision of a vitamin D supplement to all pregnant women through mother and baby clinics and health visitors may be expected to have a substantial impact in reducing risks of childbirth and perinatal mortality in Scotland [5, 20].

Summary: The recommendations made by the UK government for pregnant women need to be reconsidered urgently. The supply of Healthy Start infant vitamins needs to be reviewed to make these readily available for purchase by all mothers in Scotland. If this is done then a step-change in Scottish health may be accomplished. If it is not done then improvements in health will be delayed: current levels of ill health will continue among those with white skin while increasing levels of chronic illness may be expected among second and subsequent generations of Asians, Africans and Afro-Caribbeans who have made Scotland their home.

5. Canadians advised to take a supplement – why not Scots?

Only one in 10 Scots people take a supplement containing vitamin D and most such vitamin supplements are taken as a multi-vitamin formulation which provide a very low dose of vitamin D. Furthermore most vitamin-D-only supplements, which are available through high street chemists, also supply a rather small dose, generally not more than 400 IUs per day. Such small doses may make some small difference to health, especially for those who are surviving on a very low exposure to sunlight, but benefits of small doses have been difficult to find in large studies.

In June 2007 the Canadian Cancer Society recommended that all Canadians take 1000 IUs of vitamin D per day in autumn and winter, and in summer too if they are older or do not get much exposure to sunlight. The Canadians made the recommendation because they were impressed with trial results showing that vitamin D may prevent cancer [11].

In fact most Canadians have better opportunity to sun themselves and get vitamin D than most Scots or English. Much of Canada lies at a latitude further south than southern England and Toronto is on the same latitude as southern France. So summers are generally longer and the sun more intense for most Canadians than for people in the UK. Even though Canadian winters are severe they have continental summers with more hours of sunshine than the British Isles. So any advice to the Canadian public to get more vitamin D must apply even more to people in the UK.

However, the UK government or other UK authorities such as Cancer Research UK, the British Heart Association, Diabetes UK and other influential health charities have not yet recommended that adults, other than pregnant and nursing mothers (see above), improve their uptake of vitamin D. The main advice on sun exposure in the UK comes from Cancer Research UK, which is based in London, and although their SunSmart advice appears to be modelled on an Australian approach they have remained behind Australia when it comes to adapting their advice to what we now know are the benefits of sunshine.

Chapter 8:
Advice for individuals: how to get your vitamin D

1. Supplements – easy and reliable

Supplements are possibly the easiest way to obtain vitamin D. However there is a question concerning the best dose to take, and a small number of people with a few rare medical conditions should not take a vitamin D supplement.

The dose provided in multi-vitamin preparations and cod liver oil is much too low. A dose of 1,000 IUs per day is the minimum required to provide the majority of people with an optimum blood level. Unless a person is obtaining plenty of regular full body exposure to the sun a larger dose (2,000 IUs) is advisable to be certain of benefits [334, 374]. In Scotland regular sun exposure is not possible and so this means everyone. Tablets providing 1000 IUs of vitamin D can now be bought in the UK from Holland and Barrett, the health food store, and 500 IU tablets can be bought from Boots the chemist.

However the situation is confusing because most official advice is badly out of date. The UK government advises mistakenly that adults need no supplement unless they are housebound or cover themselves fully with clothing when outside. In fact the surveys of Hypponen and Power [24] and others [469] show that almost everyone in Scotland needs a vitamin D supplement in winter and the majority need one in the summer as well.

All authorities consider 1000 IUs of vitamin D per day to be a safe dose for any adult to take [374]. The UK Expert Group on Vitamins and Minerals has defined a "guidance level" of 1000 IU/day which is the dose of "vitamin that potentially susceptible individuals could take daily on a life-long basis, without medical supervision in reasonable safety" [470]. However guidelines in both North America and Europe have established the safe upper limit for vitamin D to be 2,000 IU per day for adults. This dose is sufficient to bring the blood level of about 85% of the population into the optimal range. However larger doses of 3,000 to 5,000 IUs would bring more people into the optimum range and may be required if full benefits are to be obtained [471, 472].

Most people living in Scotland probably need to take 5,000 IUs of vitamin D per day according to results obtained by John Aloia and colleagues from Winthrop University Hospital, Mineola, NY*. About half the Scottish population has blood levels of vitamin D below 55 nmol/L in summer and autumn and three-quarters of the population are below that level in winter and spring (Hypponen and Power). A daily dose of 5,000 IUs is needed to remedy these low levels according to Alloia and colleagues and bring them up to the optimum.

Reinhold Vieth, the Canadian expert from University of Toronto, has argued that an upper limit of 2,000 IUs per day is unreasonably low [339]. Toxicity from vitamin D in normal adults requires intakes of more than 40,000 IU per day sustained over a number of weeks or months [418]. Vieth points out that a person who receives abundant sun exposure may obtain the equivalent of an average 4,000 IU per day of vitamin D or more. Another 4,000 IU per day could be taken by mouth and there would still be a large margin of safety. A high margin of safety is also shown by a dose finding trial in which 10,000 IU per day were given to healthy men for 20 weeks without any untoward effects or any indication of excess calcium load [339].

Healthy outdoor workers

Healthy outdoor workers in the US have been found to obtain an average of 2,800 IU per day from exposure to the sun in summer [473]. Together with the vitamin D from food they obtain about 3,000 IU per day altogether. This is close to the vitamin D requirement found in a dosage trial of healthy men who were found to use from 3,000 to 5,000 IU vitamin D3 per day [474]. Vieth concludes in his review that a dose of 1000-4000 IU vitamin D per day may be sufficient, but a dose of 4,000 to 10,000 IU per day will be more certain to produce a serum level of 75-100 nmol/L in the large majority of people, a level which he describes as "desirable" [418].

On this evidence a dose of 4,000 IUs per day can be recommended to individuals, but large trials are needed to fully assess benefits and risks for the population as a whole. However risks, if any, are expected to be rare. Cannell and colleagues suggest that a dose of up to 5,000 IUs per day may be needed by people in certain risk groups, the obese, aged and/or dark skinned people, if they are to maintain adequate levels during winter [374]. Dr Cannell might

---

* Vitamin D intake to attain a desied serum 25-hydroxyvitamin D concentration. John F Aloia *et al*. Am J Clin Nutr 2008; **87**: 1952-8

well have added Scots to his list as another risk group because of the poor weather and lack of sunshine, but living in California, as he does, the special risk of living in Scotland obviously did not occur to him.

Rare contraindications

There are a few rare circumstances in which vitamin D supplements are contraindicated and should be avoided or only taken on medical advice. The most important is sarcoidosis, a condition in which tissues throughout the body, particularly lymph nodes, become inflamed and metabolise vitamin D too rapidly [475]. Others are tuberculosis, which also involves inflammation of lymph nodes, and lymphoma, a tumour of the lymph nodes. Vitamin D may actually aid recovery in tuberculosis but must be taken under medical supervision because the infected tissue may change vitamin D too rapidly into the active hormone form and upset metabolism of calcium. Anyone who suffers from hyperparathyroidism or has had bouts of hypercalcaemia should also avoid taking extra vitamin D. Hypercalcaemia may cause kidney stones and so anyone with a history of kidney stones should only take vitamin D under medical supervision with monitoring of their blood calcium.

Very rarely, a person may have one of the contraindicated conditions without it having been noticed and diagnosed or may have hyperparathyroidism which disturbs control of calcium. Such people are at risk of developing hypercalcaemia after starting a vitamin D supplement. Symptoms of hypercalcaemia include persistent nausea, vomiting, malaise, thirst, diarrhoea or constipation. Anyone who develops these symptoms in other than mild form. after starting a vitamin D supplement should consult their doctor and request a blood calcium test. Hypercalcaemia is easily treated, usually by simple oral rehydration, and does not cause long-term ill effects if it is spotted promptly.

Large doses

Vitamin D can be taken in large doses by everyone except rare individuals who have contraindications [327]. A daily dose of 4,000 IUs may be accumulated and taken safely as a single weekly dose of 28,000 IUs or a single monthly dose of 120,000 IUs according to convenience [418]. Vitamin D is stored in fat and has an effective half life in the body of between two and three months so a single monthly dose is probably as effective as a pro rata daily dose.

Two types of vitamin D are available in tablet form: cholecalciferol, also known as vitamin D3, which is the natural human molecule, and ergocalciferol or D2, which occurs mostly in plants and was in the past obtained from yeast. Ergocalciferol feeds into the same metabolic pathway as cholecalciferol but may not be so potent or so tolerable in higher doses because it is broken down in part by a different pathway. So it is recommended to prefer cholecalciferol when a choice is available [476, 477].

2. Sunbathing – the SunSafe advice

Sunbathing is the simplest and most natural way to boost vitamin D levels and if it is done safely without burning carries very little risk of skin cancer. But before going into more detail I would like to explain the experience I bring to the provision of health advice for the public. I feel it necessary to do this because my advice runs contrary to that of Cancer Research UK, a distinguished charity with a wide range of expertise.

Some 28 years ago I began with others at *The Sunday Times* newspaper to compile information about lifestyle and health. The idea, encouraged by Harry Evans, our visionary editor, was to provide a guide to healthy living. The readership of *The Sunday Times* was measured in millions and so the advice was received by millions of people. We took the job very seriously and compiled the advice in a book which we called *The Sunday Times Book of Body Maintenance* [478]. This exercise compelled me and others involved to think about what sort of advice is most valuable to the public and how best to present it. I continued to provide advice to readers when I went to *The Independent* and have continued to do so from time to time in books. I mention all this as a preface to advice that I provide here because I want to make it clear that provision of advice to the public is not a new departure for me and that I understand the serious considerations that must go into formulating it.

The SunSafe advice* (see Box 1), which I advocate here, has been carefully thought out for the reduction of risks of chronic disease from too much or too little sun. The SunSafe advice is based on a detailed appraisal of scientific evidence available in published literature. It is also conservative and reflects traditional advice given on sunlight in the UK in the past before Cancer Research UK devised its SunSmart advice with emphasis on limitation of exposure to the sun.

---

*This advice was first given in 2006 at an international conference at the House of Commons on Sunlight, Vitamin D and Health and published by Health Research Forum as Occasional Report No 2.

BOX 1: The SunSafe advice encourages safe sunbathing and safe exposure to the sun, which is our major source of vitamin D. Safe sunbathing raises vitamin D levels and so contributes to prevention of chronic disease caused by insufficient vitamin D.

The SunSafe advice is based on up-to-date scientific evidence and on the commonsense approach to sun exposure that was taken in the UK before sun avoidance was mistakenly promoted by Cancer Research UK's SunSmart advice.

The SunSafe Advice - safe and smart
1. Sunbathe safely without burning – whenever you can.
2. The middle of the day is a good time for sunbathing in the UK.
3. Remove as many clothes as you can. Start by sunbathing for 2-3 minutes each side. Gradually increase from day to day to a maximum of half an hour per side in the UK, less abroad.
4. Don't use sunscreen creams while aiming to boost vitamin D.
5. If feeling hot or uncomfortable expose a different area, cover up, move into the shade – or use sunscreen cream.
6. The face is easily over-exposed so it makes sense to wear a hat when sunbathing and when in the sun for a prolonged time.
7. When abroad, where the sun is generally stronger, expose your body for shorter times until you find out how much is safe.
8. Children benefit from sun exposure, but need guidance.
9. A tan is natural and is generally associated with good health.

3. SunSmart's mistakes – Britons told to play by Australian rules

The SunSmart advice appears to be based on an Australian programme with the same name. Australians of course need to be very careful to avoid excessive sun exposure because the sun is so much stronger there, but it has been a grave mistake to adopt similar advice for the UK. In fact Australians are now told by the Cancer Council of Australia to be sure to get some sun exposure to secure their supply of vitamin D. In the past Australian children were not allowed to play outside unless they wore a hat. The rule was simple: no hat no play. Now Australians are realizing that they need different rules for different parts of the country and in Tasmania, in the far south which gets least sun in winter, children are being told to take their hats off outside for winter play.

The SunSmart advice (see Box 2) contains no positive statements about sunlight, only negative ones. In its original form SunSmart not only failed to encourage people to expose themselves to the sun, it actively discouraged people from sun exposure of any kind. It could not be more unsuited to the British climate.

The SunSmart advice was written and approved by the UK Skin Cancer Working Party, a committee that draws its members mostly from the British Association of Dermatologists (BAD). Nine out of 17 of its committee members are from organisations concerned with skin and six other members represent government organisations. There are no representatives from other disciplines in clinical medicine. None from orthopaedics, for example, even though expert opinion concerned about bone disease has pleaded to have a voice in government advice on sun exposure since at least 1998 [373].

Negative advice of the kind given by SunSmart increases risks not only of bone disease but also many other chronic diseases caused by vitamin D insufficiency, including internal cancers. Evidence showing that cancer patients diagnosed in summer do better than those diagnosed in winter suggests that exposure to sunlight may prolong the life of cancer patients, including those with melanoma, even after the tumour is well established [479, 480]. The benefits of vitamin D that may be expected for cancer prevention are discussed in more detail in the section on cancer above.

Johan Moan, a distinguished Norwegian photobiologist, believes that the benefits of sun exposure in preventing cancer and other chronic disease far exceed any risk of skin cancer coming from sun exposure [481, 482]. He estimates that an increase in sun exposure, which might double the number of melanoma skin cancers, might save 10 times more people from dying of internal cancers. In addition it might be expected to extend the life of people with cancer and reduce the risk of heart disease, diabetes, and many other diseases. If this is the case then Cancer Research UK's SunSmart strategy risks causing much more cancer and other disease than it could ever prevent, and so the strategy must have been responsible for an untold number of cancer deaths.

CR-UK fails to inform media of changes

For this reason I have suggested that the SunSmart programme should be abandoned and replaced with a positive programme along the lines of the SunSafe advice given here [459, 483, 484]. Since I made this suggestion Cancer Research UK has modified the SunSmart message in small but significant ways (Box 2). It no longer advocates "staying in the shade between 11 am and 3 pm" but now advises the public only to "spend time in the shade between 11 am and 3 pm", and instead of telling people to "always cover up" it now advises much less categorically that people should "aim to cover up". These new exhortations obviously allow for the possibility of some sun exposure, although CR-UK still does not actually advise any sun exposure. Furthermore CR-UK has failed to inform the media or the public that there has been a change in its message and so confusion with its previous message advocating total sun avoidance remains [485].

BOX 2: The SunSmart advice from Cancer Research UK – *not recommended here.*

SunSmart – advice pre 2006
● Stay in shade between 11 am and 3 pm
● Make sure you never burn
● Always cover up
● Remember to take extra care of children
● Then use factor 15 sunscreen

More detailed instructions included the injunction to put on large amounts of suncream 20 minutes before going out into the sun, and to wear a hat. Favourite CR-UK slogans are: "Keep your shirt on" or "There's no such thing as a healthy tan".

SunSmart – change of advice in 2006
● Spend time in the shade between 11am and 3pm
● Aim to cover up with T-shirt, hat
● Then use factor 15+ sunscreen

CR-UK's message now rightly emphasises avoidance of burning but deliberate sun exposure such as sunbathing is still not encouraged. Any suggestion that there has been a change in CR-UK's message has been avoided; so now CR-UK claims disingenuously: "We never told people to avoid the sun."

Contrary to the facts, CR-UK denies that it has advised against sun exposure. In a letter responding to an article that I wrote in *The Sunday Telegraph* [486] it said: "CR-UK's SunSmart campaign has never encouraged people to avoid the sun as you suggest in your article on vitamin D but it continues to encourage people to be safe in the sun to reduce their risk of skin cancer. Our key message remains to avoid burning as sunburn is the most important risk factor in developing skin cancer."

In fact CR-UK's key message in the past was the mantra: "there is no such thing as a healthy tan". But realising that there is no scientific evidence to support this contentious catchphrase, and that a tan is inevitable for many people after even modest exposure to the sun, CR-UK has now generally ceased to repeat it. However, the mantra still stood on the website of BAD, the British Association of Dermatologists in April 2008.

Melanomas are relatively rare in dark skinned people suggesting that skin pigment may actually protect against melanoma [487]. A tan is a natural consequence of repeated exposure to the sun and does not mean that the skin has been burnt. A tan shows that a person has had some useful sun exposure and probably has a better than average level of vitamin D in the body – and so it is in fact a sign of good health. And a tan may even protect against melanoma in the same way that skin that is dark from birth is known to protect against melanoma.

SunSafe – a practical, safe approach

The SunSafe programme (see Box 1) which is recommended here provides positive guidelines for sun exposure that are based both on up-to-date evidence and common sense. This programme encourages people to expose them-selves safely to the sun. As a result, they will gain substantially more vitamin D during the summer, with consequent benefits the following winter and spring. At the same time, SunSafe warns against burning, which is the only risk of sun exposure that has been clearly linked with skin cancer [464]. The SunSafe programme provides a practical approach that codifies what many sensible British people have always done in summer.

The intensity of the sun varies greatly with the time of year, the time of day, and cloud cover while individual sensitivity to the sun depends on skin type and previous exposure. So it is not possible to give precise guidance for optimum times of exposure to the sun which may vary from minutes to hours before burning begins. For example, in the UK in September a person who does not have a sensitive skin and has had plenty of previous exposure may safely remain in the sun for an hour or more in the middle of the day, although it may be advisable to protect the face which is always in danger of over exposure.

In the British Isles we often have cloudy days in mid summer with occasional bright sunny periods that come and go quickly. On that sort of day it may be safe for someone with previous exposure and an average skin to strip to the waist for an hour or more in the middle of day – but again it may be advisable to wear a hat, otherwise the face will remain exposed much longer after the shirt has been put back on. However, in midsummer, someone with a sensitive skin and little previous exposure should only expose themselves to the sun for a few minutes on each side and gradually increase exposure over the following days and weeks.

It was not until about 1990 that professional opinion began to suggest that melanoma, the most dangerous form of skin cancer, was caused by exposure to the sun. A recent meta-analysis by Sara Gandini and colleagues has found that studies undertaken before 1990 generally found no association between sun exposure and melanoma. Whereas later studies did find an association. Gandini suggests that these later studies were influenced by biased recall of participants who knew from wide publicity that experts believed skin cancer was caused by sun exposure [464]. These later biased studies have been very influential and have determined policy for 15 or more years.

In fact the Gandini meta-analysis suggests that chronic exposure to the sun, that is regular exposure over a long period, may actually protect the skin against melanoma rather than increase the risk of this cancer. The meta-analysis shows that it is intermittent exposure to the sun that is most clearly associated with an increased risk of melanoma [464].

4. Vitamin D protects skin cells

Melanoma is more common in Scotland now than 30 years ago, and much of the increase in melanomas has occurred on areas of the body that are usually covered (chest, upper arm, upper leg and in men lower leg too) i.e. the parts that are only intermittently exposed to the sun [488]. These areas are most vulnerable to burning if exposed to the sun too rapidly at first because they lack protective melanin pigment [487].

Prolonged exposure of untanned white skin to the sun allows unprotected pigment cells (melanocytes) to be bombarded with UV rays that are likely to damage DNA and cause mutations. Vitamin D actually protects these skin cells from UV by preventing the formation of damage molecules (pyrimidine dimers) in DNA [489]. In other words vitamin D actually protects against sunburn and the risks of intermittent exposure. That is one reason why the skin is much better able to resist burning after a number of short exposures that have enabled some vitamin D to form in it. The skin also thickens and tans in response to exposure providing additional protection against harmful effects of the sun.

The middle of the day is a convenient time for many people to sunbathe. The sun is strong at this time so care must be taken not to burn. In fact the midday sun contains a higher proportion of UVB to UVA than the morning or evening sun and so more vitamin D may be obtained with reduced risk of damage to skin provided burning is avoided. Before 11am or after 3pm it is necessary to stay in the sun longer to get a good dose of vitamin D, but a proportionally larger dose of UVA, which does not make vitamin D, will be received at the same time [490].

In midsummer sun at midday, an exposure of about 20-30 minutes on each side of the body will produce a maximum quantity of vitamin D, that is between 10,000 and 20,000 IUs, [418, 491]. But take care because 20-30 minutes is longer than most people will be able to tolerate when they start sunbathing. At other times of day or other times of year when the sun is less strong a longer exposure will be necessary to produce the maximum amount of vitamin D. When the angle of the sun is less than 45° most or all of the UVB rays, which generate vitamin D in the skin, are absorbed in the atmosphere. So winter sun and the early morning and the late evening sun in summer are not effective in producing vitamin D, even when the rays are sufficiently strong to warm the skin.

There is a maximum amount of vitamin D that can be produced at one time because a chemical equilibrium occurs in the body such that the sun not only produces vitamin D but also breaks it down. However the maximum daily production of 20,000 IUs provides enough vitamin D to last from five to 10 days. It makes sense to sunbathe every day when this is possible because vitamin D is stored in body fat from which it is mobilized in the winter when the level in serum is low. Regular sunbathing will establish a good body store that may be expected to reduce the risk of winter infections including flu as well as other chronic disease.

Ann Webb and Ola Engelsen have calculated how much vitamin D may be obtained from sun exposure at various latitudes and various times of year [492]. Their calculations make many assumptions and cannot take into account all possible variations, so the calculations must be seen as illustrations rather than definitive answers. Nevertheless they show clearly that in Scotland it would be very difficult to obtain an average 4,000 IUs vitamin D per day from sun exposure alone. To do this it would necessary to obtain something like 10,000 IUs per day during the five months, April to September, which is not possible.

Nevertheless it is possible to obtain some very useful vitamin D from the sun in Scotland if there is good luck with the weather. If it is possible to sunbathe for 20 minutes in the lunch hour three days a week on average, exposing face, neck, arms, hands and legs (57% of the body surface), and in addition sunbathe once a week wearing only a bikini, then 900,000 IUs of vitamin D might be obtained from the sun between mid-April and mid-September. This can be stored in body fat and used up through the winter. Such regular sunbathing is difficult, if not impossible, for most people to achieve in Scotland. However, with a sheltered sunbathing deck and extra days of whole body sunbathing during good weather it may be possible to sunbathe twice a week, which could provide an average of more than 1,000 IUs per day and that is just about enough to take a person out of vitamin D insufficiency and avoid some long-term health risks. But for optimum health in Scotland it is advisable to take a vitamin D supplement.

White skin evolved to make the best of weak sun

In support of the SunSafe approach it is worth remembering that sunlight is a natural source of vitamin D for human beings. White skins have evolved in northern Europe where there is less sun and enable what sunlight there is to be used more effectively. This is particularly important in early spring and late summer or autumn when the sun is less strong and in a climate where brief sunny periods occur between clouds. In effect a light coloured skin extends the summer season when vitamin D can be made in skin.

It cannot be wise to suggest that a lifestyle making use of this natural source of health should be abandoned, as Cancer Research UK have done, without very clear scientific evidence to show that a change would be beneficial. Cancer Research UK and others have suggested that people in Britain remain in the shade for four hours in the middle of the day, or put on sun screen and wait 20 minutes before emerging fully clothed, with hat, into full sunlight. These suggestions should be ignored because there is no scientific evidence that such crude sun avoidance measures have any overall benefit to health while there is every reason to believe that such advice is positively harmful.

Suncream prevents burning but also prevents UVB reaching the skin and so prevents synthesis of vitamin D. So suncream should not be used at the start of sunbathing. It can be put on when your time is up and you want to end the action of UV on skin and stop burning. However, it is better to put on clothes and/or move into the shade. With some sports it is not possible to move out of the sun, when playing tennis or sailing, for example. That is when suncream is most useful.

Suncreams generally block UVB more effectively than UVA and it is now widely believed by experts that it is UVA that causes skin cancer. So suncreams may reduce the ability of skin to make vitamin D while not providing full protection against skin damage or cancer. How effective suncream is also depends on how much is used and manufacturers now encourage people to use plenty of it to achieve a complete block.

5. Sunlamps and sunbeds

Sunlamps and sunbeds expose the body to ultra violet light that not only induces a tan but also induces production of vitamin D in the skin. A five-to-10 minute exposure on a sunbed can produce more than 10,000 IUs of vitamin D which is a useful quantity providing enough for a few days [493]. However the UV light from sunlamps and sunbeds differs from sunlight in the ratio of its two components known as UVA and UVB. Light in the UVB range induces production of vitamin D but takes longer to produce a tan than UVA, which tans but does not produce any vitamin D.

A full review of sunlamps is beyond the scope of this report. However, it needs to be said that the campaign of Cancer Research UK and others against use of sunbeds has up to now been one sided, considering the possible risk of skin cancer without considering the benefits that can be gained from synthesis of extra vitamin D in skin. It has been assumed that the only benefit obtained from sunbeds is a cosmetic one when in fact there are considerable benefits from the vitamin D produced, including a feeling of well-being. Furthermore some studies have been unable to find any risk of melanoma from use of sunbeds [494].

A number of scientists have shown that exposure on sunbeds increases production of vitamin D. For example, Professor Johan Moan and colleagues have demonstrated that twice weekly exposures on a sunbed can increase the vitamin D level in the body by 40% [495]. Professor Moan goes on to consider the balance of risks and benefits from sunbed exposure, which has not often been addressed. Quoting Giovannucci's work on benefits of vitamin D in cancer prevention [496], Professor Moan and colleagues argue that moderate sunbed exposures during the winter, equivalent to a daily dose of 1500 IUs of vitamin D, would reduce total cancer deaths by 29% in the United States.

Taking the argument further, Professor Moan and colleagues calculate that at least 10 deaths from cancer might be prevented in Norway for each melanoma that is induced by sunbed sessions. He said: "Taking into account that moderate and regular sunbed exposure in winter might not necessarily lead to any large increase in the number of melanoma deaths, one should reconsider the restrictive attitude towards sun bed use."

If other benefits such as prevention of bone diseases are considered the ratio of benefit to risk from moderate sunbed use may be nearer the 2,000 to 1 level found by Lucas and discussed above [463]. Looked at in this way it seems extraordinary that such vehement objections have been raised to the use of sunbeds. This vehemence appears to have arisen from the general belief that purely commercial interests are taking advantage of frivolous cosmetic motivation and so putting lives at risk.

A feeling of well-being

As well as the general health benefits of vitamin D already outlined here, scientific trials have shown that vitamin D can induce a change of mood with a feeling of well-being [497-499]. The popularity of sunbed exposure may well be the result of this response as well as the desire for a tan which is quite rightly regarded by the public as a sign of good health. A person who has an above average tan is also likely to have an above average vitamin D level and so be healthier than most. Indeed the feeling of well-being may be a response that has an evolutionary origin – that is to encourage us to sunbathe and so be fitter in the fight for survival of the species.

The campaign against sunbeds in Scotland, and the UK generally, has led to removal of sunbeds from local authority premises such as swimming baths and there is a move to prevent their use by children. A more constructive approach would be to develop regulations that encouraged development and installation of sunlamps that maximize UVB production together with rigorous safety regulations. Once that is done it would make sense to encourage the use of sunbeds and to persuade local authorities to install them once more in their premises. In this way sunbeds could do much to raise vitamin D levels in Scotland and reduce Scotland's health deficit.

Sunlamps and sunbeds have generally been designed to produce more UVA than UVB based on the mistaken belief that UVB is more carcinogenic than UVA. This belief came from studies of squamous cell carcinoma in albino hairless mice which are now thought to have been misleading [500]. UVA is now thought by scientists to carry a greater risk of inducing melanoma, the most dangerous form of skin cancer, than UVB [501-503]. It is possible to manufacture sunlamps and sunbeds that produce a large proportion of UVB to UVA (see table).

Such lamps can provide UVB with reduced risk of harm to skin and so produce the maximum amount of vitamin D with minimum risk of melanoma. This type of lamp has been manufactured but is not in general use because it is not so effective in producing a tan. A list of these lamps that are currently available is provided in the table below. Expert independent assessment of these lamps with verification of the specifications and recommendations for optimal exposure times to obtain a suitable dose of vitamin D would be a helpful step forward.

A change in regulations and/or advice to the sunbed/sunlamp industry might change present practice so that lamps had a higher benefit to risk ratio resulting from a higher UVB to UVA ratio. Lamps that are a rich source of UVB and carry a low risk of skin cancer could make an important contribution to health in Scotland because sunlamp treatment is popular and an effective way of providing vitamin D.

So far as the current type of sunbed is concerned benefits still greatly outweigh any risk of skin cancer and so there is no firm basis for discouraging their use. Taking supplements may be a safer way of increasing vitamin D levels but many people do not like to take supplements because they consider it unnatural to take pills, or they find it is a nuisance, or they simply do not remember to take them. Other people have a problem absorbing supplements and UVB exposure is the best way for them to obtain vitamin D. For all these people sunbed treatments are the best or most convenient way to boost vitamin D levels and obtain better health.

UV lamps producing high percentage UVB

Brand	lamp type	Wattage	Length	UVB	UVA	Distributed by	Contact
Sunfit	RX Plus	100W	6ft or 180 cm	2.40%	30W	Helionova	www.helionova.co.uk
ERS	SOL-PROF ASR5-17-160	160W	6ft or 180 cm	2.50%	46W	Alpha Industries	www.alpha-industries.be
ERS	SOL-SOFT AH3-24	100W	6ft or 180 cm	1.80%	31W	Alpha Industries	www.alpha-industries.be
Philips Swift		100/160W	6ft or 180 cm	1.8-2%	30-40W	Philips	Phone +31 165 57 7011

Chapter 9:
Towards a "step-change" in Scots health

Scotland needs a "step-change" in its trajectory of health improvement if it is ever to catch up with other European nations, say Hanlon and colleagues in their report "Chasing the Scottish Effect"[1]. They go on to say: "If health is to improve, the determinants of health will have to change." At the time of their report it was not widely appreciated how important vitamin D is for health or how little vitamin D people in Scotland manage to obtain.

Vitamin D insufficiency needs to be recognised as a major determinant of the deficit in Scottish health – that is as a substantial factor causing the "Scottish Effect". Better provision of vitamin D to Scots generally could be crucial in achieving the desired step-change in Scottish health.

Individuals can do much to improve their personal vitamin D level but they need advice and encouragement to do so. To achieve a step-change in vitamin D levels of the Scottish population with the expected step-change in health that will follow requires important initiatives from the Scottish government and from leading executives in the Scottish National Health Service.

A checklist of action needed from the Scottish Government:

1. Present official UK government recommendations for daily intake of vitamin D supplements are far too low. They need to be brought up to date and based on the best international advice. The UK Scientific Advisory Committee on Nutrition (SACN) has reviewed this advice and has not recommended changes. However, SACN was not able to review all the evidence, did not take evidence from leading scientists abroad, and did not take into consideration the special circumstances of the Scottish climate that is so less well-endowed with sunlight than England. Scotland, and particularly its northern islands, receives so much less sunlight than southern England that special recommendations on intake of vitamin D supplements need to be considered for Scotland, as has been done in Canada for their northern territories above latitude 55° north. This issue requires urgent attention that has been lacking in Westminster's handling of the issue. Creation of a Scottish Scientific Committee to review policy and advice on vitamin D and sunlight would be a useful and important move.

2. New guidance is needed on sunlight/UV exposure that considers benefits as well as risks. This is very controversial, particularly in Scotland where the distinguished dermatologist Professor Rona Mackie has in the past advised against any substantial sun exposure in order to reduce the risk of skin cancer. However opinion is now changing and Professor Mackie has recently acknowledged the importance of sun exposure as a source of vitamin D. New guidance for Scots explaining how to obtain sun exposure safely without burning, as outlined here, is needed.

3. New regulations are needed that will allow suitable health claims for foods fortified with vitamin D. This will encourage manufacturers to fortify more foods because they will be able to promote them using the health claim. Health claims are now governed by EU regulations and so this will require negotiation with EU departments, which the Scottish government is able to do. However, products that are made and distributed locally could be given permission by the Scottish legislature to be fortified and to carry a suitable health claim. These items could include, for example, bread, milk, and perhaps certain fruit juices that are made locally from concentrate. Deviation from the normal EU rule may be justified because the products are not exported and Scotland lies mostly above 55 degrees North latitude.

4. People with dark skin living in Scotland are at particularly high risk of vitamin D insufficiency and of suffering associated diseases. The second generation of dark-skinned immigrant children raised in Scotland are at greater risk than their parents because they will have endured vitamin D insufficiency since birth. If nothing is done to remedy their low levels of vitamin D they may be expected to suffer a high incidence of diseases associated with low D. New recommendations and ready availability of suitable supplements are needed together with a new initiative building on the previous experience in Glasgow in the 1960s-1980s.

5. Doctors in the UK lack a suitable range of vitamin D supplements available for prescribing. This could be overcome by relatively simple administrative measures that allowed rapid approval of new vitamin D products on the basis of purity and absorption capability without demanding full clinical trials. New vitamin D3 (cholecalciferol) products providing 2,000 IUs, 14,000 IUs, and 60,000 IUs to be taken daily, weekly or monthly are needed. The Scottish government is in the fortunate position where it could make any necessary administrative changes, or create new law, to facilitate this without having to wait for Westminster.

6. Another approach would be to enable rapid approval of European vitamin D products to allow their sale in the UK without having to undergo extensive and irrelevant testing procedures designed for new drugs. Vitamin D products presently available in Europe could be approved after simple tests to assure the purity and absorbability of the product. The Scottish government could, if necessary, create new law to allow special import of vitamins. The German vitamin D supplement known as Vigantol Oil sold by Merck of Darm-stadt has been found to be particularly useful by some UK doctors but at present is only available after special arrangements for prescription to individuals are satisfied. And a convenient 50,000 IU tablet of vitamin D3 is made in New Zealand which could be imported immediately without delay if facilitated by the Scottish government.

7. Scientific trials of vitamin D for treatment and prevention of chronic disease need to be funded. Scotland is an ideal place for such trials because the incidence of disease caused at least in part by vitamin D is so high.

8. Special consideration needs to be given to advice on vitamin D for sports people. Present knowledge suggests that an increase in vitamin D levels of sports people could increase strength and fitness and reduce the risk of certain injuries in those who have inadequate levels.

9. Much could be gained from an international meeting of doctors and scientists expert in vitamin D insufficiency and associated disease together with Scottish public health experts. I hope that the Scottish government might be prepared to fund such a meeting.

Chapter 10:
Sir Richard Doll and vitamin D
– with a note on James Watson

1. Influence of a non-significant trend

In 1950 Sir Richard Doll published the first study showing that smoking could cause not only lung cancer but also heart attacks and emphysema. At first the work was treated with great scepticism that was encouraged by the vested interests of the tobacco industry. Sir Richard himself stopped smoking but it was many years before he convinced others of the dangers of tobacco. Eventually his work became the foundation for official reports on the risks of smoking.

During the final years of his life Sir Richard developed another interest that again influenced his personal habits. Sir Richard had shown in a study, undertaken with Daksha Trivedi and Kay Tee Khaw, that vitamin D reduces fractures in people over 65 [327]. The study also showed a reduction in mortality in the subjects who took vitamin D. Sir Richard was impressed by this trend, even though the reduction in mortality did not reach statistical significance. He believed his findings suggested a general beneficial effect of vitamin D, not just an effect on bone. And he started to take a monthly vitamin D tablet providing the equivalent of about 1,000 IUs per day.

Sir Richard Doll

Later work has indeed confirmed Sir Richard's belief that his observations on mortality were a clue to something significant. A meta-analysis by Philippe Autier of the International Agency for Research in Cancer in Lyons and Sara Gandini of the European Institute of Oncology in Milan have since shown that taking a vitamin D supplement does reduce mortality – by 7% over a period of about six years [10].

In the year before his death, Doll was reviewing the literature on vitamin D and sunlight. The study he had undertaken with Trivedi and Khaw was intended to be a pilot project, and Doll still hoped to obtain funding for a larger trial that would examine a wider range of possible benefits. Sir Richard read my report *Sunlight Robbery* and was interested in the large number of associations between vitamin D insufficiency and chronic disease that are outlined in it. He told me he believed many of the associations were probably true but added, with a statistician's prescience, that it was unlikely that all were true. He concluded by saying that it was clear vitamin D is very important for good health.

2. Courageous change of mind

In the summer of 2004 I went with Julian Peto to talk to Sir Richard about vitamin D and the possibility of under-taking a trial of the vitamin for prevention of chronic disease. We also discussed the beneficial effects of exposure to the sun and the lack of scientific evidence to back up the current recommendations of government to avoid exposure in the middle of the day in the UK. Sir Richard had courageously changed his mind on the subject of sun exposure influenced by his own findings and in part too, I believe, by my report *Sunlight Robbery*.

As chairman of the UK Advisory Group on Non-ionising Radiation (AGNIR) he had signed off a report of the National Radiological Protection Board (NRPB) which states that casual exposure to the sun in the UK provides people with sufficient vitamin D [22]. This mistaken belief that what you get is what you need remained a foundation stone of official policy on sunlight in the UK until very recently. The "casual exposure assertion", as we might call it, cannot be true because the majority of people in the UK have sub-optimal levels of vitamin D in both winter and summer and the sun is our major source of the vitamin [5].

When Sir Richard looked further into the evidence he realised that the "casual exposure assertion" could not be supported scientifically. However, he did not want his revised opinion to be made public until he had formally notified the NRPB. So following discussion during our visit, Sir Richard said he must telephone Professor Tony Swerdlow, the presiding chairman of AGNIR, to report his change of view. He was anxious to be courteous and did not wish Swerdlow to hear of his change of view for the first time in a newspaper article.

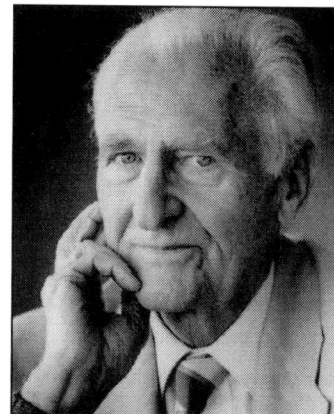

Sir Richard felt that the subject of vitamin D had not had the attention it deserved from scientists and that a great deal more needed to be achieved. As we departed he said: "This isn't difficult science. We should have answers."

Since that meeting in 2004 scientific understanding of vitamin D has burgeoned and we have many more answers although, as always in science, as many questions remain. We even have evidence now suggesting that vitamin D may diminish the risk of lung cancer caused by smoking [97, 504]. Sadly Sir Richard did not live long enough to see much of these new developments. He died in July 2005 at the grand old age of 92. If he could have had another lifetime available to him I believe he would have made major contributions to research on vitamin D

After our meeting Sir Richard wrote to Julian Peto in October 2004 as follows: "I have been corresponding with Oliver Gillie over the possible benefits of vitamin D and have, of course, known him otherwise for some time. I am most impressed with the way he has collected and presented the vitamin D evidence. He is, in my opinion, a serious scientist who knows a great deal about the subject of his present interest. There is, I think, a lot to be done in this field which may affect national policy."

I had known Sir Richard for many years, having first met him when I was medical correspondent of the *Sunday Times* writing about the dangers of smoking. Among other matters he had shown interest in an article I wrote explaining for the first time how the last four British Kings suffered and died from smoking diseases. On another occasion he had been angered when I wrote something about asbestos and cancer that he was not ready to disclose.

I reprint Sir Richard's generous reference here because my role as both journalist and scientist sometimes attracts criticism. Publication of my earlier report "Sunlight Robbery" without formal peer review meant for some that it could be dismissed without consideration. Cancer Research UK, for example, did not respond to it or even acknowledge receipt of it until I sent a copy to each of their trustees. So I offer here Sir Richard Doll's words as evidence of my bonafides and as an endorsement of my scientific purpose. I very much hope that this report on Scotland's health will receive serious consideration.

3. James Watson, DNA and vitamin D

In the early 1950s James Watson together with Francis Crick and Maurice Wilkins discovered the structure of DNA, hailed as the most important biological discovery of the 20th century. In 2008, some 50 years later, Watson called together a meeting of some of the world's most distinguished scientists to celebrate his 80th birthday and among other matters talk about how to live longer. Watson, like Doll, was taking a small aspirin daily but recently had started to take vitamin D as well.

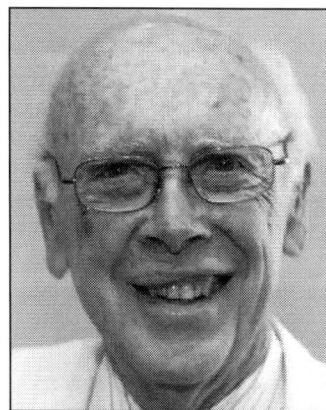

James Watson

Ironically, an awareness of the role of vitamin D in prevention of cancer began some 25 years before, but Watson, like most scientists, had no inkling of its importance until recently. Our understanding of the vital place of vitamin D in human health owes little to modern genetics, the science that burgeoned out of Watson's discovery of DNA structure. Many millions of dollars and pounds in government support were spent on "high-tech" genetics with astounding success, leading to many major discoveries.

During the same period comparatively little money was spent in "low-tech" studies of vitamin D. The vital role of the vitamin in chronic disease was largely established by means of classical clinical and physiological investigations, classical biochemical investigation of metabolic pathways, and the orphan science of epidemiology. The work began 100 years ago with investigations of rickets and now, after the work of thousands of scientists, has led to one of the major discoveries of modern medicine – perhaps just in time to extend the life of Nobel Laureate, James Watson.

Chapter 11:
Finding the trail – how this began

I hope that this book will start a debate that will lead to a reassessment of public policy on vitamin D and sunlight, and perhaps ultimately to a step-change in Scottish health. It has not been easy to persuade scientists, doctors and policy makers who have become committed to an established public health policy on sunlight and vitamin D to think again and question their assumptions. There has been a distinct reluctance to address the difficult issues involved.

Some may think it is presumptuous of a person best known as a journalist and writer to attempt to argue a case with experts who have spent a lifetime studying their subject. But most of the scientists I know, while maintaining an energetic scepticism, have been prepared to consider the case for sunlight and vitamin D on its merits, and increasing numbers are persuaded of its importance.

Even so, some will ask why a writer is meddling in matters that are more often left to the wisdom of expert committees. It may help to explain something of the background to this book and how I became involved in these issues. In the following two chapters I offer a miscellany of information explaining the origin of this project, which has absorbed much of my time for the last five or six years.

1. Sunlight Robbery

How it all started: For many years I followed scientific work exploring the origins and causes of schizophrenia. In the 1970s to 1990s one school of thought, which is still influential, considered the major cause of schizophrenia would be found in the genes. Theirs was the orthodox view and their dogma was often expressed in the form "schizophrenia is 90% genetic". My own view, as someone who had studied advanced genetics for my doctorate, was that these researchers were using faulty methodology and failing to take account of serious discrepancies that made their observations inconsistent with a largely genetic explanation of the disease.

These ideas were shared with a small minority of those interested in the cause or causes of schizophrenia. I thought I might explore the ideas in a book. In fact this has since been done with great expertise by Jay Joseph in his important book called *The Gene Illusion* which puts the misguided optimism and dogma of psychogeneticists to shame [505]. As it happened I was already pursuing a different line when Jay Joseph's book appeared. I had begun to look closely at research on environmental factors that were known to be associated in some way with schizophrenia.

This led me to research showing that birthdays of schizophrenic people clustered in spring and early summer. Endeavouring to understand what might cause this clustering of birthdays I looked at other diseases, multiple sclerosis and diabetes type 1, which showed a similar clustering of birthdays. I thought I might find another disease that might provide a model or at least help in some way to explain the processes involved in causation of schizophrenia.

I started to collect as much information as I could on seasonal effects in disease and searched for explanations. At first I thought that folic acid deficiency, well known then as the cause of neural tube and brain defects, might occur seasonally and cause an abnormal development of the brain leading to schizophrenia.

It was Dr Kay Tee Khaw, the distinguished epidemiologist who worked with Sir Richard Doll on vitamin D supplementation, who suggested to me that vitamin D might be a common factor causing seasonal influences on disease. About the same time I became aware of the work of Dr John McGrath at the Queensland Centre for Mental Health Research in Australia, which showed further possible links between schizophrenia and vitamin D insufficiency. Dr McGrath's work has gone from strength to strength and includes a demonstration that insufficient vitamin D given to rat mothers during pregnancy causes brain damage in the offspring. However, this work is still in some ways at an early stage and remains controversial so I have not pursued it in this book.

My own research in the scientific literature went on to examine all the diseases that were associated in some way with vitamin D insufficiency, including surrogate effects on vitamin D uptake such as latitude, altitude, skin colour and urban/rural differences. I was astounded to find that there were so many diseases that appeared to be associated with differences in vitamin D and/or exposure to the sun or its surrogates. At this time in 2002 or 2003 the importance of vitamin D as a hormone that activates genes in virtually every organ or tissue of the body was known only to a tiny group of interested scientists. Consideration of the consequences for public health policy had not begun and few, if any, were willing to challenge the conventional wisdom of cancer experts who were telling the public to avoid the sun.

I considered that if so many diseases are caused by insufficient vitamin D and vitamin D insufficiency is so widespread then there may be something wrong with accepted policy on sunlight. This led me to write *Sunlight Robbery: Health benefits of sunlight are denied by current public health policy in the UK*. Then, in order to spread these ideas further I set up Health Research Forum, as described below, to promote evidence based public health policy.

It occurred to me early in my research that Scotland had a special problem with vitamin D insufficiency and the diseases that it brings. I assembled much of the research for this book some four years ago but could not find the time to write it. But I was determined not to let the project drop for three reasons. Of all countries in the world Scotland probably illustrates better than any other the dire effects of vitamin D insufficiency on the population. Yet until very recently this seems to have gone completely unrecognised in Scotland. I also felt that I had a debt to repay to Scotland for the nine important years I spent at Edinburgh University. Finally I thought that the newly independent Scottish government might be more inclined to listen than Westminster and would have the will to take steps to remedy the situation.

2. Scotland – a personal note

I have many links with Scotland that have helped me in writing this book. My affection for Scotland, together with the hope that the new Scottish government will be interested in taking up the issues described here, has kept me going.

I was raised on Tyneside but spent almost 10 years in Scotland as a student at Edinburgh University and loved the country and the people. As an undergraduate I lived at 22 West Preston Street where my two landladies, Miss Paterson and Miss Fairbairn, provided me with a small room and meals. Finnan haddie and kippers (oily fish rich in D) were a regular item in the high tea served at 6 .00pm on the dot. Miss Paterson was fond of saying that Geordies were "economy Scotsmen", an expression I took to heart. I can see her saying it now with a twinkle in her eye as she stirred the hot coals with a poker to get more heat from the fire. Her *bons mots* could have many meanings, but I felt it was a good description of my relationship with, what was for me at that time, my adopted country.

However, my links with Scotland go much further back than that. My family came originally from Berwickshire and the culture persisted down the generations. That did not just mean oatcakes with heather honey or kippers for tea. Kippers were a common enough item in North Shields where we lived. It also meant that words like bairn, muck and clarts were part of my father's everyday vocabulary.

So writing this report on Scottish health has been a work of honour and perhaps duty too: a duty because I feel that it identifies an urgent problem that is remediable. When the necessary provisions are made by the Scottish government and other authorities, as they must be sooner or later, big improvements in the health of people in Scotland may be expected. And it is an honour because I feel privileged to be able to point to something which I hope and believe is likely to make a big difference to people in Scotland.

I would like here to thank my father, John Calder Gillie, who has been an inspiration to me in undertaking this work. He was, if ever there was one, a true economy Scotsman, raised largely on Tyneside but educated in part in Scotland by a Presbyterian dominee. In his latter years we discussed this work on sunlight and vitamin D and he gave me much encouragement. He was born in 1906 and, having taken a great interest in science and health all his life, he knew about the discovery of vitamin D. He had witnessed how amazed the world had been to learn early in the last century that vitamin D was synthesised by the effects of sun on skin.

Like many of his generation who loved the outdoors my father would take off his shirt and enjoy the benefit of sunlight whenever he had an opportunity. The climate of the Northumberland coast, like that of Scotland, is not generous with sunshine. Even so I remember him when he was 94 changing into his shorts to mow the lawn and sit in the garden in the sun. Sometime in the late 1940s or early 1950s he bought a UV lamp and me and my two brothers stripped off, put on special goggles and sat with him in front of the lamp to absorb the rays and make vitamin D. It was an impressive ritual, sitting round the lamp with its strange colours and surreal glow.

My father and his sisters, like many other children of his time, were given cod liver oil everyday. It was a traditional tonic, especially perhaps for Scots because of Scotland's long-held connection with fishing. Nobody then knew that cod liver oil was rich in vitamin D and omega 3 fatty acids. My father also ate kippers and herring regularly, and fish of all kinds, which were always available fresh in North Shields. He enjoyed walking and walked to work every day. These habits, together with an abstemious nature, may account for him living to the age of 96.

I wish I could tell my father what I have found out about Scottish health. I am sure he would be very interested. I miss him greatly and offer this work as a tribute to him.

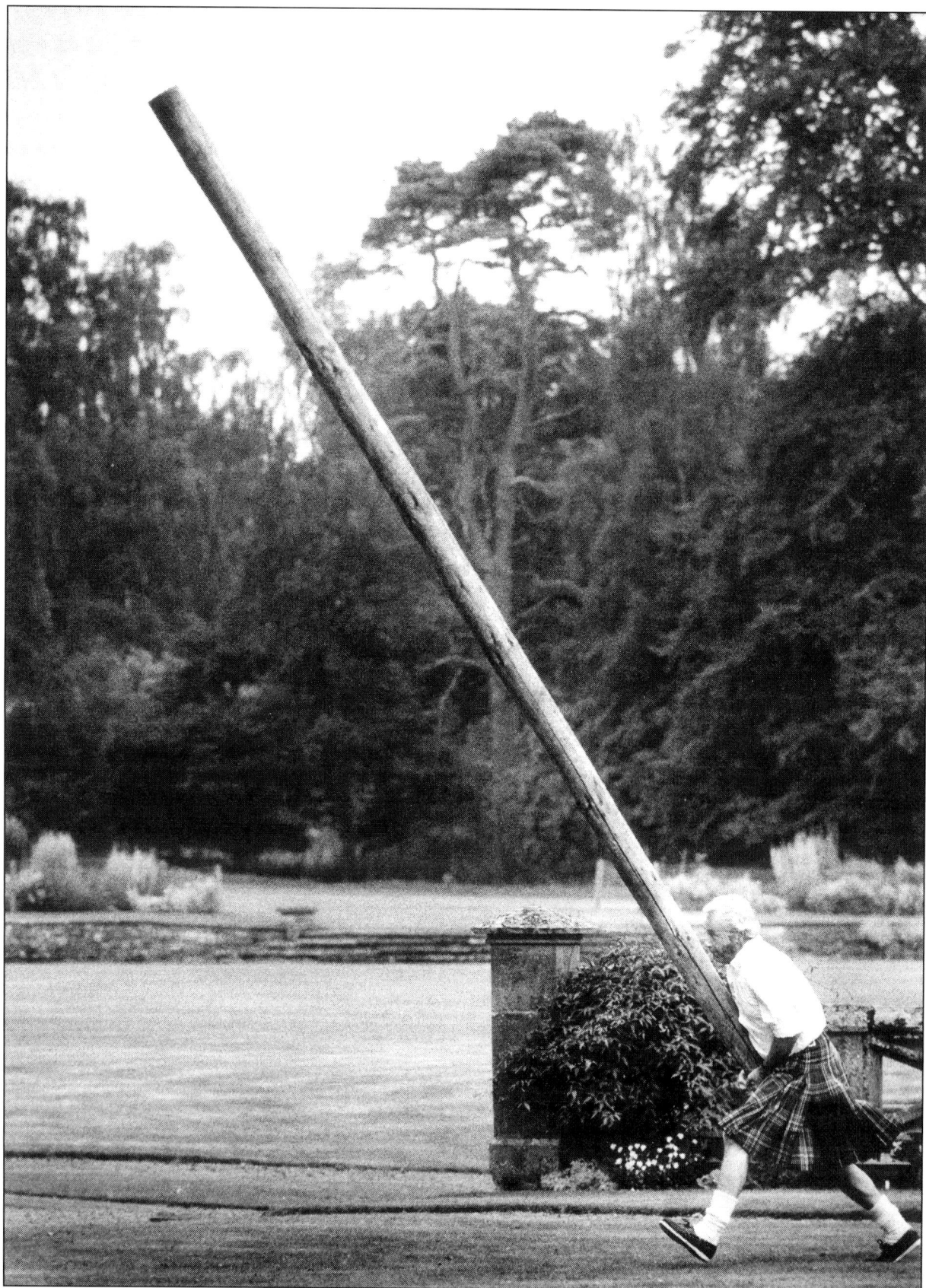

A possible Scot - Oliver Gillie tosses the caber.
Picture : Brian Harris

Chapter 12:
For the record

1. Health Research Forum: report of activities

The aim of Health Research Forum (HRF) is to develop an up-to-date public health policy based on scientific evidence. It takes time, often decades, for new scientific ideas to be accepted and assimilated, first into the general body of scientific knowledge and finally into policy. We want to reduce this time to the minimum so that benefits of research leading to a better understanding of health will become available without delay. We hope to provide policy makers with better information on which to base national health policy and individuals with better information on which to base choices about their lifestyles.

To achieve these ends I have lobbied government, briefed journalists, staged a conference, published reports, and interested researchers in starting trials. This book on Scotland's Health Deficit is the third report to be published by Health Research Forum.

Health Research Forum advisors

Director and founder:
Oliver Gillie

Scientific advisors:
Moray Campbell, Department of Pharmacology and Experimental Therapeutics, Roswell Park Cancer Institute, Buffalo, NY

William Grant, Sunlight, Nutrition, and Health Research Center (SUNARC) San Francisco

Michael Holick, Boston University, School of Medicine, Boston

Julian Peto, London School of Hygiene and Tropical Medicine, London

Joy Townsend, London School of Hygiene and Tropical Medicine, London

Reinhold Vieth, Department of Nutritional Sciences, University of Toronto and Mt Sinai Hospital, Toronto, Canada

Advisors on production and publicity:

Michael Crozier – Editorial Director of Crozier Associates Ltd, formerly of *The Independent* and *The Times*

Jim Anderson – freelance journalist, formerly of *The Sunday Telegraph*

Sunlight Robbery

The first report *Sunlight Robbery* [457] was published in 2004 and proved to be effective in raising questions about advice on sunlight given by the government and by Cancer Research UK. *Sunlight Robbery* obtained publicity in the media, raised the profile of issues around sunlight and health and persuaded many people who had been avoiding sunlight to change their habits and seek the sun while taking care to avoid burning.

Sunlight Robbery also proved to be influential abroad, particularly in Australia where advice to the public on sun exposure has since changed fundamentally. Many Australians have very low levels of vitamin D in their serum, even those living in sub-tropical Queensland. My report became available at a time when some Australians felt that the "slip, slap slop" health initiative which recommended avoidance of the sun needed a radical reappraisal.

Jeremy Laurance, health editor of *The Independent*, was told when he visited Australia that *Sunlight Robbery* was influential in stoking controversy concerning vitamin D in Australia and in assisting a reassessment of entrenched health advice on sunlight. Australians are no longer advised to avoid the sun completely, but are now told to expose their bodies to the sun for a time before putting on suncreams and protective clothing.

The influence of *Sunlight Robbery* also extended to Europe with its translation into French and presentation for consideration to the French government's health department.

House of Commons conference

In 2005 Health Research Forum (HRF) organised a conference at the House of Commons under the aegis of Ian Gibson MP who acted as chairman. Some 120 people attended, including many scientists, doctors, government officers and other policy makers. Papers presented at the conference were published by HRF as a report with the title *Sunlight, Vitamin D and Health* [506]. In the report I suggested that new advice on sun exposure was needed and recommended sunbathing while taking care not to burn. The argument advanced at the conference was later published in full under my name in the British Journal of Dermatology [507].

In response to these criticisms Cancer Research UK, which is the principle source of government advice on sun exposure, broadened their advisory committee to include a greater number of people. CR-UK also changed its advice to the public and no longer recommends people to "always cover up" and to "stay in the shade between 11am and 3pm" as they did for many years as part of their SunSmart programme. This advice was clearly wrong because outside these midday hours the sun is relatively weak in the UK and is not capable of making much vitamin D in the skin. As explained in detail above, anyone following CR-UK's advice and covering up, using suncream and staying in the shade during these hours, would get little or no vitamin D so greatly increasing their risk of chronic disease including cancer.

New advice from CR-UK

Now CR-UK's advice is less categorical. Early in 2007 CR-UK began to say: *"aim to cover up"* and *"spend time in the shade between 11am and 3pm"*. The change is small but all the more significant for that. CR-UK obviously felt the need to move away from the extreme position it held previously. However CR-UK has failed to publicise its change of advice and continued throughout the summer of 2007 to provide the old advice on parts of its website. As a result the old advice continued to be advocated by the media during the summer of 2007 and 2008. CR-UK's stealthy change suggests that it may have been uneasy and did not wish to explain reasons for the shift.

In March 2006 Ian Gibson MP arranged for me to meet Caroline Flint, secretary of state responsible for public health. I asked her to take several initiatives to improve vitamin D levels in the country. Following our meeting the Scientific Advisory Committee on Nutrition (SACN) was asked by her to consider issues around vitamin D. SACN published a report *Update on Vitamin D* in 2007 [158]. Regrettably SACN was not able to take sufficient time to examine the literature on vitamin D and chronic disease in detail. Nor did SACN consider in any detail what degree of sun exposure is needed in the UK to obtain an optimum level of vitamin D. As a result they made very conservative recommendations.

Now an official vitamin D campaign

Nevertheless the Department of Health has launched what it has called a "vitamin D campaign" and seems to have changed its position slightly in favour of sun exposure. The Department now suggests "it takes only 15 minutes exposure of arms, head and shoulders in the sun each day during the summer months to make enough vitamin D for good health". This is a welcome increase on the Department's previous suggestion that casual exposure was sufficient or that it was only necessary to expose hands and face to the sun for 10 minutes two or three times a week. Baring of the shoulders is suggested for the first time in this new advice.

However, these new recommendations are not based on a full consideration of assumptions involved but simply follow outdated guidelines as has been done in the past by CR-UK and its advisors [459]. The method used has been examined in some detail above in the section "Longer sun exposures needed for optimum vitamin D".

A proper calculation of the sun exposure necessary to produce optimum amounts of vitamin D in the skin in the UK could be made. I have had extensive discussion with Dr Dianne Godar of the FDA in Rockville, Maryland, on the way that this could be done. I discussed this approach in a meeting with Dr Jill Meara and others at the Health Protection Agency in September 2006 but as yet I know of no progress using this approach in the UK.

In our meeting with Caroline Flint I specially requested that something should be done urgently to provide children with a vitamin D supplement. Until about 1998 the government supplied vitamin D to children in a formulation known as NHS infant vitamin drops but these were withdrawn. In the autumn of 2007 government started to provide a vitamin D supplement as part of the Healthy Start programme but few children benefit from this initiative and the programe has up to now been a failure as I have described in an article in *The Daily Telegraph* [93]. Health Research Forum continues to lobby for the Healthy Start children's vitamins to be made available on sale to all children and not just to those on benefits and those belonging to ethnic minorities.

Clinical trials

I first discussed a clinical trial with Julian Peto in 2004 and this led to the meeting with Sir Richard Doll, described above. The meeting ended with Doll telling us that he would write to the Medical Research Council to raise the possibility of obtaining funds for a large trial. This initiative came to no immediate conclusion and ended when Sir Richard Doll died.

Our next approach was to Dr Jane Armitage of the Oxford Clinical Trials Unit. Dr Armitage was very interested but fully committed to other projects and so unable to take on full time involvement in a trial at that time. The possibility of a small pilot trial was discussed and I prepared a first draft of an application for funds.

I then introduced Julian Peto to Dr Adrian Martineau, who had already established experience of research in vitamin D and tuberculosis. Over a period of more than a year we discussed the design of a large trial with Dr Irwin Nazareth, director of the MRC General Practice Research Framework. This finally culminated in November 2007 in an application to Cancer Research UK for funds for a pilot trial using a two monthly dose of 120,000 IU sent by post. This application was turned down and we are currently applying for government funds.

Advanced plans for another pilot trial have been made by a group in Scotland led by Professor Aziz Sheikh. This trial is more of a dose ranging study aimed at finding the best dose of vitamin D to use in a larger trial. The initiative for the trial began with an Edinburgh GP, Dr Helga Rhein. Dr Rhein got in touch with me following a radio broadcast because she had a number of Asian patients in her practice who were very deficient in vitamin D. We corresponded over several months and I introduced her to the scientific literature on vitamin D. I was then able to help her assemble the team of Scottish trialists by introducing her to Dr Barbara Boucher and Dr Elina Hypponen.

Heart risk

Vitamin D has not yet gained wide acceptance as a risk factor for heart disease among doctors and scientists concerned about cardiac problems. For example, the National Heart Forum monitors information in specialist journals and other media about risk factors for heart disease but does not include vitamin D among the subjects it follows. I therefore compiled a dossier documenting emerging evidence showing that vitamin D insufficiency can be an important factor in heart disease, which I presented to the NHF governing committee. The committee discussed it and agreed that a meeting on vitamin D and heart disease would be organised by NHF in 2008.

2. A note on methodology: investigative review

I began this work some four or five years ago when I was researching *Sunlight Robbery*, but was unable to start writing until autumn 2007. The approach I have used in this report is the same as that used in *Sunlight Robbery* [457]. Research has involved multiple interrogation of databases, mostly PubMed, using words such as: Scotland, mortality, cancer, heart disease, diabetes, prevalence, incidence, Scottish effect, etc. In *Sunlight Robbery* I used the term "investigative review" to describe the method used and explained it as follows:

"This method of inquiry has developed from my own experience in both scientific and journalistic investigations. I call this method of research 'investigative review' to distinguish it from narrative review, which may have a marked individual slant, and systematic review, which may restrict itself to answering certain predetermined questions.

"Investigative review, on the other hand, is based on the idea that we do not always know the best questions to ask at the beginning of an inquiry, and that certain assumptions may need to be tested against the literature before we know the best questions to put. An important part of the process is to highlight incorrect assumptions that are widely held about a body of data, and to gather scattered evidence that question existing ideas and may support a new interpretation . . .

"Despite its importance, research on vitamin D has not been fashionable* and so its wider relevance has been largely overlooked. An investigative review aims to gather together such scattered evidence and, in this case, consider its relevance to national policy. The narrative in an investigative review consists then of a theme giving an account of what has been discovered and the evidence for it and may present a *prime facie* case for consideration of a new interpretation of evidence or a change of policy."

3. Brief biography

Oliver Gillie is a scientist and journalist with 25 years experience working for national newspapers in the UK. During the last six years he has been engaged in researching environmental causes of chronic disease, in particular the effects of vitamin D deprivation. This has led to the publication of *Sunlight Robbery* – a report which shows how health benefits of sunlight are denied to the public by current government policy, and to the foundation of the non-profit Health Research Forum which is dedicated to investigating the evidence base for public health policy.

Oliver Gillie has won 16 awards for his journalism, including British Science Writer of the year (three times) and British National Press Awards (four times). The Queen awarded him the Royal Jubilee medal for his work in science and health journalism.

His work on sunlight and vitamin D has been recognised by his peers with awards: an article in *The Independent* newspaper was selected as best health feature by the Medical Journalists' Association of the UK (2005). It was also chosen as best science feature in a national newspaper by the Association of British Science Writers (2005). His report *Sunlight Robbery* has been commended (MJA book awards 2005).

During his time as medical correspondent of *The Sunday Times* and medical editor of *The Independent* Oliver Gillie wrote about the major changes in medicine from heart transplantation to the eradication of smallpox. While medical editor of *The Independent* he started the Health Page, which was an immediate success and was copied by all the other national quality dailies.

Oliver Gillie is a former chairman of the Medical Journalists' Association and a trustee of the Caroline Walker Trust, the campaigning charity that has set new standards for school food. He has BSc and PhD degrees from Edinburgh University where he studied developmental biology and genetics under Professor C.H.Waddington, the distinguished geneticist and embryologist. He also worked at the National Institute for Medical Research in Mill Hill, London, under Sir Peter Medawar and has published several scientific papers.

Oliver Gillie has two daughters and two sons. He lives with his wife Jan Thompson, managing editor of *The Observer*, in north London.

---

* The situation has changed since I first wrote this. Output of research on vitamin D has grown greatly over the last few years but still it remains unknown to many clinical doctors and public health specialists, or its importance is not fully appreciated by them.

References

1. Hanlon, P., et al., *Why is mortality higher in Scotland than in England and Wales? Decreasing influence of socioeconomic deprivation between 1981 and 2001 supports the existence of the 'Scottish Effect'.* J Public Health (Oxf), 2005. **27** (2): p199-204.

2. SCF, *The Possible Scot – making healthy public policy*, S. Stewart, ed., 1999, Scottish Council Foundation: Edinburgh.

3. *Nutrition and Bone Health.* 1998, Committee on Medical Aspects of Food Policy (COMA), Department of Health, UK: London. p41-43.

4. Gallacher, S., et al., *Prevalence of vitamin D inadequacy in Scottish adults with vertebral fragility fractures.* Curr Med Res Opin, 2005. **21** (9): p1355-62.

5. Hypponen, E., et al., *Does vitamin D supplementation in infancy reduce the risk of pre-eclampsia?* Eur J Clin Nutr, 2007. **61** (9): p1136-9.

6. Burleigh, E. and Potter, J., *Vitamin D deficiency in outpatients: a Scottish perspective.* Scott Med J. 2006. **51** (2): p27-31.

7. Thane, C.W., et al., *Plasma phylloquinone (vitamin K1) concentration and its relationship to intake in a national sample of British elderly people.* Br J Nutr, 2002. **87** (6): p615-22.

8. Grant, W. and Holick, M., *Benefits and requirements of vitamin D for optimal health: a review.* Altern Med Rev, 2005. **10** (2): p94-111.

9. Giovannucci, E., *Can vitamin D reduce total mortality?* Arch Intern Med, 2007. **167**: p1709-1710.

10. Autier, P. Gandini, S., *Vitamin D supplementation and total mortality.* Arch Intern Med, 2007. **167** (16): p1730-37.

11. Lappe, J.M., et al., *Vitamin D and calcium supplementation reduces cancer risk: results of a randomized trial.* Am J Clin Nutr, 2007. **85** (6): p1586-91.

12. *Improving health in Scotland: The challenge.* 2003, Scottish Executive.

13. Hughes, A.M., et al., *Sun exposure may protect against Hodgkin lymphoma: a case-control study.* Int. J. Cancer, 2004. **112** (5): p865-71.

14. *Delivering for Health 2005*, Scottish Executive

15. *Towards a healthier Scotland – a white paper on health.* 1999, Scottish Office.

16. *Health Inequalities in the New Scotland.* 2002, Glasgow: Health Promotion Policy Unit and Public Health Institute, Scotland.

17. Langley, R.G., Sober, A.J., *A clinical review of the evidence for the role of ultraviolet radiation in the etiology of cutaneous melanoma.* Cancer Invest, 1997. **15** (6): p561-7.

18. Health Protection Scotland. Scottish Executive, 2007.

19. Scottish Public Health Observatory, in NHS Scotland and ISD Scotland. 2007.

20. Bodnar, L.M., et al., *Maternal vitamin D deficiency increases the risk of preeclampsia.* J Clin Endocrinol Metab, 2007. **92** (9): p3517-22.

21. *Building a better Scotland – 2004 Spending Review*, in *Scottish Executive.* 2004.

22. *Health effects from ultraviolet radiation.* Documents of the NRPB, ed. A.J. Swerdlow. Vol. 13. 2002, Chilton, Oxfordshire: National Radiological Protection Board

23. Gies, P., et al., *Global solar UV index: Australian measurements, forecasts and comparison with the UK.* Photochemistry and Photobiology, 2004. **79** (1): p32-39.

24. Hypponen, E., Power, C., *Hypovitaminosis D in British adults at age 45y: nationwide cohort study of dietary and lifestyle predictors.* Am J Clin Nutr, 2007. **85** (3): p860-8.

25. Dawson-Hughes, B., et al., *Estimates of optimal vitamin D status.* Osteoporos Int., 2005. **16** (7): p. 713-6.

26. Brody, H. personal communication to O. Gillie, 2007: London.

27. Hutchison, R., *Report on dietaries of Scotch agricultural labourers.* Trans. Highl. Agric. Soc. Scot., 1868. **4th ser., 2**: p1.

28. Roberts, C., *The unnatural history of the sea. The past and future of humanity and fishing.* 2007, London: Gaia Thinking.

29. Grant, W., Holick, M., *A review of evidence supporting the role of vitamin D in reducing the risk of non-skeletal diseases.* American Journal of Clinical Nutrition, 2004

30. Grant, W., *Roles of solar ultraviolet radiation and vitamin D in human health and how to obtain*

vitamin D. Expert Review of Dermatology, 2007.

31. Grant, W., *Roles of solar ultraviolet radiation and vitamin D in human health and how to obtain vitamin D.* Expert Review Dermatol., 2007. **2** (5): p563-77.

32. Tavera-Mendoza, L.E. and White, J.H.,*Cell defenses and the sunshine vitamin.* Sci Am, 2007. **297** (5): p62-5 68-70, 72.

33. Zittermann, A. and Schleithoff, S.S., Koerfer, R., *Putting cardiovascular disease and vitamin D insufficiency into perspective.* British Journal of Nutrition, 2005. **94**: p483-492.

34. Zittermann, A., *Vitamin D and disease prevention with special reference to cardiovascular disease.* Prog Biophys Mol Biol., 2006. **92** (1): p39-48.

35. Scaife, A.R., *et al., Maternal intake of antioxidant vitamins in pregnancy in relation to maternal and fetal plasma levels at delivery.* Br J Nutr, 2006. **95** (4): p771-8.

36. Das, G., *et al., Hypovitaminosis D among healthy adolescent girls attending an inner city school.* Arch Dis Child, 2006. **91** (7): p569-72.

37. Davey Smith, G., *et al., Ethnic inequalities in health: a review of UK epidemiological evidence.* Critical Public Health, 2000. **10**: p375-408.

38. Bhopal, R., *et al., Variation in all cause and cardiovascular mortality by country of birth in Scotland, 1997-2003.* Scottish Medical Journal, 2007. **52** (4): p5-10.

39. Weiler, H., *et al., Vitamin D deficiency and whole-body and femur bone mass relative to weight in healthy newborns.* Cmaj, 2005. **172** (6): p757-61.

40. Carstairs, V. and Morris, R., *Deprivation: explaining differences in mortality between Scotland and England and Wales.* BMJ, 1989. **299**: p886-889.

41. Walsh, W., Talbot, M., Hanlon, P.,*The aftershock of deindustrialisation. Trends in mortality in Scotland and other parts of post-industrial Europe.* 2008, Glasgow Centre for Population Health: Glasgow.

42. Cannegieter, S., *et al., Understanding the health of Scotland's population in an international context. Part II Comparative mortality analysis.* 2003, London School of Hygiene and Tropical Medicine.

43. Lawlor, D., *et al.,The association between temperature around the time of birth and coronary heart disease: findings from the British women's heart and health study.* abstract. Pediatric Research, 2003. **53** (6): p20A.

44. Scragg, R., *Sunlight, Vitamin D and Cardiovascular Disease, in Calcium Regulating Hormones.* C.A. Avioli, ed.. 1995, CRC Press.

45. Scragg, R., *Seasonality of cardiovascular disease mortality and the possible protective effect of ultra-violet radiation.* International Journal of Epidemiology, 1981. **10**: p337-341.

46. Scragg, R., *et al., Myocardial infraction is inversely associated with plasma 25-hydroxyvitamin D3 levels: a community based study.* International Journal of Epidemiology, 1990. **19** (3): p559-563.

47. Scragg, R., Khaw, K.T., *Life-style factors associated with winter serum 25-hydroxyvitamin D levels in elderly adults.* Age and Ageing, 1995. **24**: p271-275.

48. Scragg, R., Khaw, K.T., Murphy, S., *Effect of winter oral vitamin D3 supplementation on cardiovascular risk factors in elderly adults.* Eur J Clin Nutr, 1995. **49** (9): p640-6.

49. Elford, J., *et al., Migration and geographic variations in ischaemic heart disease in Great Britain.* Lancet, 1989. **1 (8634)**: p343-6.

50. Morris, R., *et al., Geographic variation in incidence of coronary heart disease in Britain: the contribution of established risk factors.* Heart, 2001. **86** (3): p277-83.

51. Morris, R., *et al., North-south gradients in Britain for stroke and CHD: are they explained by the same factors?* Stroke, 2003. **34**: p2604-2609.

52. Rostand, S., *Ultraviolet light may contribute to geographic and racial blood pressure differences.* Hypertension, 1997. **30**: p150-6.

53. Forman, J.P., *et al., Plasma 25-hydroxyvitamin D levels and risk of incident hypertension.* Hypertension, 2007. **49** (5): p1063-9.

54. Judd, S., *et al., Optimal vitamin D status attenuates the age-associated increase in systolic blood pressure in white Americans: results from the third National Health Nutrition Examination Survey.* Am J of Clin Nut., 2008. **87** (1): p136-141.

55. Delmas, P.D., *et al., Effect of monitoring bone turnover markers on persistence with risedronate treatment of postmenopausal osteoporosis.* J Clin Endocrinol Metab, 2007. **92** (4): p1296-304.

56. Wannamethee, S., *et al., Migration within Great Britain and cardiovascular disease: early life and adult*

See note

environmental factors. Int J Epidemiol., 2002. **31** (5): p1054-60.

57. Freathy, R.M., *et al., Type 2 diabetes TCF7L2 risk genotypes alter birth weight: a study of 24,053 individuals.* Am J Hum Genet, 2007. **80** (6): p1150-61.

58. MacPherson, A. and Bacso, J., *Relationship of hair calcium concentration to incidence of coronary heart disease.* The Science of the Total Environment, 2000. **255**: p11-19.

59. Melamed, M., *et al.* (2008) *Serum 25-hydroxyvitamin D levels and the prevalence of peripheral arterial disease. Results from NHANES 2001 to 2004.* Arteriosclosis, Thrombosis amd Vascular Biology

60. Snijder, M.B., *et al., Vitamin D status and parathyroid hormone levels in relation to blood pressure: a population-based study in older men and women.* J Intern Med, 2007. **261** (6): p558-65.

61. Krause, R., *et al., Ultraviolet B and blood pressure.* Lancet, 1998. **352**: p709-10.

62. Pfeiffer, M., *et al., Effects of a short term vitamin D and calcium supplementation on body sway and secondary hyperparathyroidism in elderly women.* Journal of Bone and Mineral Research, 2000. **15**: p1113-8.

63. Lind, L., *et al., Reduction of blood pressure by treatment with alphacalcidol.* Acta Med Scand, 1988. **223**: p211-217.

64. Prospective Studies Collaboration. *Age-specific relevance of usual blood pressure to vascular mortality: a meta-analysis of individual data for one million adults in 61 prospective studies.* Lancet, 2002. **360**: p.1903-13.

65. Collins, R. and MacMahon, S., *Blood pressure, antihypertensive drug treatment, and the risks of stroke and of coronary heart disease.* Br Med Bull, 1994. **50**: p272-98.

66. Progress, C.G., *Randomised trial of aperindopril-based blood pressure-lowering regimen among 6105 individuals with previous stroke or transient ischaemic attack.* Lancet, 2001. **358**: p1033-1041.

67. Marniemi, J., *et al., Dietary and serum vitamins and minerals as predictors of myocardial infarction and stroke in elderly subjects.* Nutr Metab Cardiovasc Dis, 2005. **15** (3): p188-97.

68. Poole, K.E., *et al., Reduced vitamin D in acute stroke.* Stroke, 2006. 37(1): p243-5.

69. Turin, T., *et al., Higher stroke incidence in the spring season regardless of conventional risk factors. Takashima Stroke Registry, Japan, 1988-2001.* Stroke, 2008. published online before print 7.2.08.

70. Stewart, S., *et al., Heart failure and the aging population: an increasing burden in the 21st century?* Heart, 2003. **89** (1): p49-53.

71. McDonagh, T., *et al., Symptomatic and asymptomatic left-ventricular systolic dysfunction in an urban population.* Lancet, 1997. **350**: p829-833.

72. Davies, M., *et al., Prevalence of left-ventricular systolic dysfunction and heart failure in the Echocardiographic Heart of England screening study: a population based study.* Lancet, 2001. **358**: p439-444.

73. Wang, T., *et al., Vitamin D deficiency and risk of cardiovascular disease.* Circulation, 2008. **117**: p503-511.

74. Zittermann, A., *Vitamin D and disease prevention with special reference to cardiovascular disease.* Prog Biophys Mol Biol., 2006. **92** (1): p39-48.

75. Michos, E.D. and Blumenthal, R.S., *Vitamin D supplementation and cardiovascular disease risk.* Circulation, 2007. **115** (7): p827-8.

76. Zittermann, A., Schleithoff, S., Koerfer, R., *Vitamin D insufficiency in congestive heart failure: why and what to do about it?* Heart Fail Rev, 2006. **11** (1): p25-33.

77. Zittermann, A., *Vitamin D in preventive medicine: are we ignoring the evidence?* Br J Nutr, 2003. **89** (5): p552-72.

78. Zittermann, A., *et al., Low vitamin D status: a contributing factor in the pathogenesis of congestive heart failure?* J Am Coll Cardiol, 2003. **41** (1): p105-12.

79. Vieth, R., *et al., The urgent need to recommend an intake of vitamin D that is effective.* Am J Clin Nutr, 2007. **85** (3): p649-50.

80. Zittermann, A., Schleithoff, S.S. and Koerfer, R., *Vitamin D insufficiency in congestive heart failure: why and what to do about it?* Heart Fail Rev, 2006. **11** (1): p25-33.

81. Weber, K., *Furosemide in the long-term management of heart failure: the good, the bad, and the uncertain.* J Am Coll Cardiol., 2004. 44(6): p1308-10.

82. Cannell, J.J., *et al., Epidemic influenza and vitamin D.* Epidemiol Infect, 2006. **134** (6): p1129-40.

83. Wong, M., *et al., Vitamin D derivatives acutely reduce endothelium-dependent contractions in the aorta of the spontaneously hypertensive rat.* Am J Physiol Heart Circ Physiol, 2008.

84. Sugden, J., *et al., Vitamin D improves endothelial function in patients with Type 2 diabetes mellitus and low vitamin D levels.* Diabet Med, 2008. **25** (3): p320-5.

85. Andrews, R., et al., *New-onset heart failure due to heart mucle disease in childhood. A prospective study in the United Kingdom and Ireland.* Circulation, 2007. published online December 17.

86. Sane, D., *Vitamin D deficiency: An under-diagnosed cause of pediatric heart failure?* Circulation, 2008. published on line February 29.

87. Lipshultz, S., et al., *The incidence of pediatric cardiomyopathy in two regions of the United States.* New Engl J Med, 2003. **348**: p1647-1655.

88. Burch, M., Reply to Dr Sane. Circulation, 2008.

89. Naiya, S., et al., *Hypocalcaemia and vitamin D deficiency: an important, but preventable cause of life threatening infant heart failure.* Heart, 2008. Heart: p. Aug 9. epub ahead of print.

90. Henederson, J., et al., *The importance of limited exposure to ultraviolet radiation and dietary factors in the aetiology of Asian rickets: a risk factor model.* Quarterly Journal of Medicine, 1987. New series **63** (241).

91. Towbin, J., et al., *Incidence, causes, and outcomes of dilated cardiomyopathy in children.* JAMA, 2006. **296** (15): p1867-76.

92. Daubeny, P., et al., *National Australian Cardiomyopathy Study. Clinical features and outcomes of childhood dilated cardiomyopathy: results from a national population based study.* Circulation, 2006. **114** (24): p2671-8.

93. Gillie, O., *Why vitamin D is so vital,* in Daily Telegraph. 2007: London.

94. Garland, C., et al., *The role of vitamin D in cancer prevention.* American J Public Health, 2006. **96** (2): p9-18.

95. Andlin-Sobocki, P., et al., *Cost of disorders of the brain in Europe.* European Journal of Neurology 2005. **12** (s): p1-27.

96. Gillis, C., Hole, D., Hawthorne, V., *Cigarette smoking and male lung cancer in an area of very high incidence-II Report of a general population cohort study in the West of Scotland.* J Epidemiology and Community Health, 1988. **42**: p44-48.

97. Mohr, S.B., et al., *Could ultraviolet B irradiance and vitamin D be associated with lower incidence rates of lung cancer?* J Epidemiol Community Health, 2008. **62** (1): p69-74.

98. Kimlin, M., et al., *Does a high UV environment ensure adequate vitamin D status?* Journal of Photochemistry and Photobiology B: Biology, 2007. **89**: p139-147.

99. Jogn, E., GG, et al., *Sun exposure, vitamin D receptor gene polymorphisms, and breast cancer risk in a multi-ethnic population.* Am J Epidemiol, 2007.

100. Giovannucci, E., *Vitamin D and cancer incidence in the Harvard cohorts.* Ann Epidemiol, 2008.

101. Boyle, I.T., *Vitamin D and ultra violet radiation.* Scott Med J, 1980. **25** (1): p1-3.

102. *Results of the first round of a demonstration pilot of screening for colorectal cancer in the United Kingdom.* UK Colorectal Cancer Screening Pilot Group. BMJ, 2004. **329**: p133-135.

103. Grant, W., Garland, C., *A critical review of studies on vitamin D in relation to colorectal cancer.* Nutr Cancer, 2004. **48** (2): p115-23.

104. Holick, M., *Does sunscreen block the skin's ability to make vitamin D? If so, how can I get enough of this vitamin without raising my risk of skin cancer?* Health News, 2002. **8** (7): p12.

105. Hughes, A.M., et al., *Sun exposure may protect against Hodgkin lymphoma: a case-control study.* Int. J. Cancer, 2004. **112** (5): p865-71.

106. Giovannucci, E., *The epidemiology of vitamin D and cancer incidence and mortality: A review (United States).* Cancer Causes and Control, 2005. **16**: p83-95.

107. Boffetta, P., et al., *Exposure to ultrAviolet radiation and risk of malignant lymphoma and multiple myeloma – a multicentre European case-control study.* International Journal of Epidemiology, 2008.

108. Grant, W.B., Garland, C.F., Gorham, E.D., *An estimate of cancer mortality rate reductions in Europe and the US with 1,000 IU of oral vitamin D per day.* Recent Results Cancer Res, 2007. **174**: p225-34.

109. Scragg, R., *Vitamin D, sun exposure and cancer: A review prepared for the Cancer Society of New Zealand.* 2007, Cancer Society of New Zealand: New Zealand.

110. Ahn, J., et al., *Serum vitamin D concentration and prostate cancer risk: A nested case-control study.* Journal of the National Cancer Institute., 2008.

111. Holick, M.F., *The vitamin D epidemic and its health consequences.* J Nutr, 2005. **135** (11): p2739S-48S.

112. Holick, M., *Evolution and function of vitamin D.* Recent Results in Cancer Research, 2003. **164**: p3-28.

113. Holick, M.F., *Vitamin D: important for prevention of osteoporosis, cardiovascular heart disease, type 1 diabetes, autoimmune diseases, and some cancers.* South Med J, 2005. **98** (10): p1024-7.

114. Morrissey, P.E., Flynn, M.L., Lin, S., *Medication non-compliance and its implications in transplant recipients.*

Drugs, 2007. **67** (10): p1463-81. *See note*

115. van Dam, R.M., *et al., Diet and basal cell carcinoma of the skin in a prospective cohort of men.* Am J Clin Nutr, 2000. **71** (1): p135-41.

116. Eyles, D., *et al., Vitamin D3 and brain development.* Neuroscience, 2003. **118**: p41-53.

117. Hayes, C.E., Cantorna, M.T. and DeLuca, H.F., *Vitamin D and multiple sclerosis.* Proc Soc Exp Biol Med, 1997. **216** (1): p21-7.

118. Poon, A.H., *et al., Association of vitamin D receptor genetic variants with susceptibility to asthma and atopy.* Am J Respir Crit Care Med, 2004. **170** (9): p967-73.

119. Lucas, R.M. and Ponsonby, A.L. *Ultraviolet radiation and health: friend and foe.* Med J Aust, 2002. **177** (11-12): p594-8.

120. Cantorna, M., *Vitamin D and its role in immunology: Multiple sclerosis, and inflammatory bowel disease.* Progress in Biophysics and Molecular Biology., 2006. **92** (1): p60-64.

121. Cantorna, M.T., *Vitamin D and autoimmunity: is vitamin D status an environmental factor affecting autoimmune disease prevalence?* Proc Soc Exp Biol Med, 2000. **223** (3): p230-3.

122. Cantorna, M.T., *et al., Vitamin D status, 1,25-dihydroxyvitamin D3, and the immune system.* Am J Clin Nutr, 2004. **80** (6 Suppl): p1717S-20S.

123. Liebmann, P., *et al., Melatonin and the immune system.* Int Arch Allergy Immunol, 1997. **112**: p203-211.

124. DeMarco, P.J. and Constantinescu, F., *Does vitamin D supplementation contribute to the modulation of osteoarthritis by bisphosphonates? Comment on the article by Carbone* et al. Arthritis Rheum, 2005. **52** (5): p1622-3; author reply 1623.

125. Demko, C.A., *et al., Use of indoor tanning facilities by white adolescents in the United States.* Arch Pediatr Adolesc Med, 2003. **157** (9): p854-60.

126. Jacobson, D.L., *et al., Epidemiology and estimated population burden of selected autoimmune diseases in the United States.* Clin Immunol Immunopathol, 1997. **84** (3): p223-43.

127. Cooper, C.R., *et al., Preferential adhesion of prostate cancer cells to bone is mediated by binding to bone marrow endothelial cells as compared to extracellular matrix components* in vitro. Clin Cancer Res, 2000. **6** (12): p4839-47.

128. Hill, A., *The Environment and Disease: Association or Causation.* Proceedings of the Royal Society of Medicine, 1965. **58**: p295-300.

129. Do, J., *et al., Effects of vitamin D on expression of Toll-like receptors of monocytes from patients with Behçet's disease.* Rheumatology, 2008. **47** (6): p840-848.

130. Adorini, L., *Intervention in autoimmunity: the potential of vitamin D receptor agonists.* Cell Immunol., 2005. **233**: p115-124.

131. Harel, M., Shoenfeld, Y., *Predicting and preventing autoimmunity, myth or reality?* Ann NY Acad Sci, 2006. **1069**: p322-345.

132. Arnson, Y., H. Amital, and Y. Shoenfeld, Vitamin D and autoimmunity: new aetiological and therapeutic considerations. Ann Rheum Dis, 2007. **66**(9): p1137-42.

133. Willer, C., *et al., Timing of birth influences multiple sclerosis susceptibility: the Canadian Collaborative Study Group.* British Medical Journal, 2005. **330** (7483): p120.

134. Forbes, D., *Oral vitamin D3 supplementation reduced fractures in community dwelling elderly people.* Evid Based Nurs, 2003. **6** (4): p113.

135. Shepherd, D. and Downie, A., *A further prevalence study of multiple sclerosis in northeast Scotland.* J Neurol Neurosurg Psychiatry, 1980. **43**: p310-315.

136. Poskanzer, D., *et al., Multiple sclerosis in the Orkney and Shetland Islands 1: Epidemiology, clinical factors, and methodology.* J Epidemiology and Community Health, 1980. **34**: p229-239.

137. Alikasifoglu, A., *et al., Neonatal hyperparathyroidism due to maternal hypoparathyroidism and vitamin D deficiency: a cause of multiple bone fractures.* Clin Pediatr (Phila), 2005. **44** (3): p267-9.

138. Shepherd, D. and Summers, A., *Prevalence of multiple sclerosis in Rochdale.* J Neurol Neurosurg Psychiatry, 1996. **61**: p415-17.

139. Swingler, R.J. and Compston, D., *The prevalence of multiple sclerosis in south east Wales.* J Neurol Neurosurg Psychiatry, 1988. **51**: p.520-4.

140. Mumford, C., *et al., Multiple sclerosis in the Cambridge health district of East Anglia.* J Neurol Neurosurg Psychiatry, 1992. **55**: p877-82.

141. Williams, G., Harrold, J.A. and Cutler, D.J., *The hypothalamus and the regulation of energy homeostasis:*

lifting the lid on a black box. Proc Nutr Soc, 2000. **59** (3): p385-96.

142. Roberts, M.H., *et al., The prevalence of multiple sclerosis in the Southampton and South West Hampshire Health Authority.* J Neurol Neurosurg Psychiatry, 1991. **54** (1): p55-9.

143. Rice-Oxley, M., Williams, E.S., Rees, J., *A prevalence survey of multiple sclerosis in Sussex.* J Neurol Neurosurg Psychiatry, 1995. **58**: p27-30.

144. Goldacre, M., *et al., Skin cancer in people with multiple sclerosis: a record linkage study.* J Epidemiology Community Health, 2004. **58**: p142-4.

145. Albertazzi, P., *et al., Hyperparathyroidism in elderly osteopenic women.* Maturitas, 2002. **43** (4): p245-9.

146. Holmoy, T., *A Norse contribution to the history of neurological diseases.* Eur Neurol, 2006. **55** (1).

147. Ascherio, A. and Munger, K., *Environmental risk factors for multiple sclerosis. Part 1: The role of infection.* Ann Neurol, 2007. **61**: p288-299.

148. Chaudhuri, A., *Why we should offer routine vitamin D supplementation in pregnancy and childhood to prevent multiple sclerosis.* Med Hypotheses, 2005. **64** (3): p608-18.

149. van der Mei, I.A., *et al., Past exposure to sun, skin phenotype, and risk of multiple sclerosis: case-control study.* BMJ, 2003. **327** (7410): p316.

150. Vassalo, L., M. Elian, M., Dean, G, *Multiple sclerosis in southern Europe. II: Prevalence in Malta in 1978.* J Epidemiology Community Health, 1978. **33**: p111-3.

151. Hammond, S.R., English, D.R., McLeod, J.G., *The age-range of risk of developing multiple sclerosis: evidence from a migrant population in Australia.* Brain, 2000. **123** (Pt 5): p968-74.

152. Hammond, S.R., *et al., The epidemiology of multiple sclerosis in three Australian cities: Perth, Newcastle and Hobart.* Brain, 1988. **111** (Pt 1): p1-25.

153. Freedman, D., Dosemeci, M., McGlynn, K., *Sunlight and mortality from breast, ovarian, colon, prostate, and non-melanoma skin cancer: a composite death certificate based case-control study.* Occup Environ Med, 2002. **59**: p257-62.

154. Sandyk, R., Awerbuch, G.I., *Multiple sclerosis: relationship between seasonal variations of relapse and age of onset.* Int J Neurosci, 1993. **71** (1-4): p147-57.

155. Embry, A., *Vitamin D supplementation in the fight against multiple sclerosis.* J Orthomolec Med, 2004.

156. Doilu-Hanninen, M., *et al., A longitudinal study of serum 25-hydroxyvitamin D and intact parathyroid hormone levels indicate the importance of vitamin D and calcium homeostasis regulation in multiple sclerosis.* Journal of Neurology, Neurosurgery, and Psychiatry, 2008. **79**: p152-157.

157. Ebers, G.C., *Environmental factors and multiple sclerosis.* Lancet Neurol, 2008. **7** (3): p268-77.

158. *Update on Vitamin D. Position statement by the Scientific Advisory Committee on Nutrition.* (SACN), 2007: London.

159. Munger, K., *et al., Vitamin D intake and incidence of multiple sclerosis.* Neurology, 2004. **62**: p60-5.

160. Black, H.S., *et al., Evidence that a low-fat diet reduces the occurrence of non-melanoma skin cancer.* Int J Cancer, 1995. **62** (2): p65-9.

161. Brown, S.J., *The role of vitamin D in multiple sclerosis.* Ann Pharmacother, 2006. **40** (6): p1158-61.

162. Orton, S.M., *et al., Sex ratio of multiple sclerosis in Canada: a longitudinal study.* Lancet Neurol, 2006. **5** (11): p932-6.

163. Metcalfe, M., Baum, J., *Incidence of insulin dependent diabetes in children aged under 15 years in the British Isles during 1988.* BMJ, 1991. **302**: p443-447.

164. Rangasami, J.J., *et al., Rising incidence of type 1 diabetes in Scottish children, 1984-93. The Scottish Study Group for the Care of Young Diabetics.* Arch Dis Child, 1997. **77** (3): p210-3.

165. Green, A., Patterson, C.C., *Trends in the incidence of childhood-onset diabetes in Europe 1989-1998.* Diabetologia, 2001. **44 Suppl 3**: pB3-8.

166. EURODIAB, *Vitamin D supplement in early childhood and risk of Type I (insulin-dependent) diabetes mellitus.* Diabetologia, 1999. **42**: p51-54.

167. Blom, L.,Persson, L.A., Dahlquist, G., *A high linear growth is associated with an increased risk of childhood diabetes mellitus.* Diabetologia, 1992. **35** (6): p528-33.

168. Dahlquist, G., Bennich, S.S., Kallen, B., *Intrauterine growth pattern and risk of childhood onset insulin dependent (type I) diabetes: population based case-control study.* BMJ, 1996. **313**.

169. Waldhor, T., Schober, E., Rami, B., *The Austrian Diabetes Incidence Study Group. Regional distribution of risk for childhood diabetes in Austria and possible association with body mass index.* Eur J Paediatr, 2003. **162**: 380-384.

170. Larsson, C.L., Johansson, G.K., *Young Swedish vegans have different sources of nutrients than young omnivores.* J Am Diet Assoc, 2005. **105** (9): p1438-41.

171. Hypponen, E., et al., *Infant feeding, early weight gain, and risk of type 1 diabetes. Childhood Diabetes in Finland (DiMe) Study Group.* Diabetes Care, 1999. **22** (12): p1961-5.

172. The EURODIAB substudy 2 Study Group. *Rapid early growth is associated with increased risk of childhood type 1 diabetes in various European populations.* Diabetes Care, 2002. **25**: p1755-1760.

173. Tenconi, M., et al., *Major childhood infectious diseases and other determinants associated with type 1 diabetes: a case-control study.* Pavia T1DM Registry Group. Acta Diabetol., 2007. **44** (1): p14-9.

174. Zipitis, C., Akobeng, A., *Vitamin D supplementation in early childhood and risk of type 1 diabetes: a systematic review and meta-analysis.* Arch. Dis Child, 2007.

175. Green, A., Gale, E.A., Patterson, C.C., *Incidence of childhood-onset insulin-dependent diabetes mellitus: the EURODIAB ACE Study.* Lancet, 1992. **339** (8798): p905-9.

176. Songini, M., et al., *The Sardinian IDDM study: 1. Epidemiology and geographical distribution of IDDM in Sardinia during 1989 to 1994.* Diabetologia, 1998. **41** (2): p221-7.

177. Meloni, T., et al., *IDDM and early infant feeding. Sardinian case-control study.* Diabetes Care, 1997. **20** (3): p340-2.

178. Daaboul, J., et al., *Vitamin D deficiency in pregnant and breast-feeding women and their infants.* J Perinatol., 1997. **17** (1): p10-4.

179. Pettifor, J., *Nutritional rickets: deficiency of vitamin D, calcium, or both?* Amer J Clin Nutr, 2004. **80** (6S): p1725S-1729S.

180. Levy-Marchal, C., C. Patterson, Green, A., *Variation by age group and seasonality at diagnosis of childhood IDDM in Europe. The EURODIAB ACE Study Group.* Diabetologia, 1995. **38** (7): p823-30.

181. Glatthaar, C., et al., *Diabetes in Western Australian children: descriptive epidemiology.* Med J Aust, 1988. **148**: p117-123.

182. Cannell, J.J., V.R., Umhau, J.C., Holick, M.F., Grant, W.B., Madronich, S., Garland, C.F., Giovannucci, E., *Epidemic influenza and vitamin D.* Epidemiol Infect., 2006. **134** (6): p1129-40.

183. Soedamah-Muthu, S., et al., *All-cause mortality rates in patients with type 1 diabetes mellitus compared with a non-diabetic population from the UK general practice research database, 1992-1999.* Diabetologia, 2006. **49** (4): p660-6.

184. Janghorbani, M., et al., *Systematic review of type 1 and type 2 diabetes mellitus and risk of fracture.* Am J Epidemiol, 2007. **166** (5): p495-505.

185. Pittas, A.G., et al., *The role of vitamin D and calcium in type 2 diabetes. A systematic review and meta-analysis.* J Clin Endocrinol Metab, 2007. **92** (6): p2017-29.

186. Boucher, B.J., *Inadequate vitamin D status: does it contribute to disorders comprising syndrome 'X'?* British Journal of Nutrition, 1998. **79**: p315-327.

187. Boucher, B.J., et al., *Glucose intolerance and impairment of insulin secretion in relation to vitamin D deficiency in east London Asians.* Diabetologia, 1995. **38** (10): p1239-45.

188. Ruohola, J.P., et al., *Association between serum 25(OH)D concentrations and bone stress fractures in Finnish young men.* J Bone Miner Res, 2006. **21** (9): p1483-8.

189. McLean, G., Guthrie, B., Sutton, M., *Differences in the quality of primary medical care of CVD and diabetes across the NHS: evidence from the quality and outcomes framework.* BMC Health Services Research, 2007. **7** (74).

190. Hannawi, S., et al., *Atherosclerotic disease is increased in recent onset rheumatoid arthritis: a critical role for inflammation.* Arthritis Research and Therapy, 2007. **9** (6).

191. Als, O.S., Riis, B., Christiansen, C., *Serum concentration of vitamin D metabolites in rheumatoid arthritis.* Clin Rheumatol, 1987. **6** (2): p238-43.

192. Aguado, P., et al., [*High prevalence of vitamin D deficiency in postmenopausal women at a rheumatology office in Madrid. Evaluation of 2 vitamin D prescription regimens*]. Med Clin (Barc), 2000. **114** (9): p326-30.

193. Kroger, H., Penttila, M., Alhava, E., *Low serum vitamin D metabolites in women with rheumatoid arthritis.* Scand J Rheumatol, 1993. **22**: p172-7.

194. Patel, S., et al., *Association between serum vitamin D metabolite levels and disease activity in patients with early inflammatory polyarthritis.* Arthritis Rheum, 2007. **56** (7): p2143-9.

195. Oelzner, P., et al., *Relationship between disease activity and serum levels of vitamin D metabolites and PTH in rheumatoid arthritis.* Calcified Tissue International 1998. **62**: p193-198.

196. Oelzner, P., et al., Relationship between soluble markers of immune activation and bone turnover in post-menopausal women with rheumatoid arthritis. Rheumatology (Oxford), 1999. **38** (9): p841-7.

197. Tetlow, L.C., et al., Vitamin D receptors in the rheumatoid lesion: expression by chondrocytes, macrophages, and synoviocytes. Ann Rheum Dis, 1999. **58** (2): p118-21.

198. Jones, S.M., Bhalla, A.K., Osteoporosis in rheumatoid arthritis. Clin Exp Rheumatol, 1993. **11** (5): p557-62.

199. Hansen, M., et al., Bone loss in rheumatoid arthritis. Influence of disease activity, duration of the disease, functional capacity, and corticosteroid treatment. Scand J Rheumatol, 1996. **25** (6): p367-76.

200. Andjelkovic, Z., et al., Disease modifying and immunomodulatory effects of high dose 1 alpha (OH) D3 in rheumatoid arthritis patients. Clin Exp Rheumatol, 1999. **17** (4): p453-6.

201. Dottori, L., D'Ottavio, D., Brundisini, B., Calcifediol and calcitonin in the therapy of rheumatoid arthritis. A short term controlled study (in Italian). Minerva Medicine, 1982. **73**: p3033-3040.

202. Rohult, J., Jonson, B., Effects of large doses of calciferol on patients with rheumatoid arthritis. Scandinavian Journal of Rheumatology, 1973. **2**: p173-176.

203. Barthel, H.R., Scharla, S.H., [Benefits beyond the bones — vitamin D against falls, cancer, hypertension and autoimmune diseases]. Dtsch Med Wochenschr, 2003. **128** (9): p440-6.

204. Cantorna, M., Hayes, C., DeLuca, H., 1,25-dihydroxycholecalciferol inhibits the progression of arthritis in murine models of human arthritis. J Nutr, 1998. **128**: p68-72.

205. Frediani, B., et al., [Study of vitamin D status of rheumatoid arthritis patients. Rationale and design of a cross-sectional study by the osteoporosis and metabolic bone diseases study group of the Italian Society of Rheumatology (SIR)]. Reumatismo, 2006. **58** (4): p314-8.

206. Svendsen, A.J., et al., Relative importance of genetic effects in rheumatoid arthritis: historical cohort study of Danish nationwide twin population. BMJ, 2002. **324** (7332): p264-6.

207. Hameed, K., et al., The prevalence of rheumatoid arthritis in affluent and poor urban communities of Pakistan. Br J Rheumatol, 1995. **34** (3): p252-6.

208. Harkness, E., et al., Is musculoskeletal pain more common now than 40 years ago? two population-based cross-sectional studies. Rheumatology, 2005. **44**: p890-895.

209. Lau, E., et al., Low prevalence of rheumatoid arthritis in the urbanized Chinese of Hong Kong. J Rheumatol, 1993. **20** (7): p1133-7.

210. Cimmino, M.A., et al., Prevalence of rheumatoid arthritis in Italy: the Chiavari Study. Ann Rheum Dis, 1998. **57** (5): p315-8.

211. Kauppinen-Makelin, R., et al., A high prevalence of hypovitaminosis D in Finnish medical in and out patients. Intern Med, 2001. **249**: p559-63.

212. Alamanos, Y., Voulgari, P.V., Drosos, A.A., Incidence and prevalence of rheumatoid arthritis, based on the 1987 American College of Rheumatology criteria: a systematic review. Semin Arthritis Rheum, 2006. **36** (3): p182-8.

213. Drosos, A., Rheumatoid arthritis: clinical pciture and therapeutic considerations. Autoimmunity Reviews. **3 Suppl 1**: pS20-S22.

214. Salvarani, C., et al., Extra-articular manifestations of rheumatoid arthritis and HLA antigens in Northern Italy. J Rheumatol., 1992. **19**: p242-6.

215. Gare, B., Juvenile arthritis – Who gets it, where and when? A review of current data on incidence and prevalence. Clin Exp Rheumatol, 1999. **17**: p367-374.

216. Forseth, K.O., [Treatment of rheumatic patients in a warm climate abroad]. Tidsskr Nor Laegeforen, 2007. **127** (4): p449-52.

217. Wiles, N., et al., Estimating the incidence of rheumatoid arthritis: trying to hit a moving target? Arthritis Rheum, 1999. **42** (7): p1339-46.

218. Webb, A., et al., Correction of vitamin D deficiency in elderly long-stay patients by sunlight exposure. J Nutritional Medicine, 1990. **1**: p201-7.

219. Stojanovic, R., et al., Prevalence of rheumatoid arthritis in Belgrade, Yugoslavia. Br J Rheumatol, 1998. **37** (7): p729-32.

220. Power, M.L., et al., The role of calcium in health and disease. Am J Obstet Gynecol, 1999. **181** (6): p1560-9.

221. Pusch, K., et al., Gull eggs – food of high organic pollutant content? J Environ Monit, 2005. **7** (6): p635-9.

222. Serhan, E., et al., Prevalence of hypovitaminosis D in Indo-Asian patients attending a rheumatology clinic. Bone, 1999. **25**: p609-11.

223. Harris, S., Dawson-Hughes, B., Seasonal changes in plasma 25-hydroxyvitamin D concentrations of young

American black and white women. American J Clinical Nutrition, 1998. **67**: p1232-1236.

224. Plotinikoff, G. and B. Quigley, Prevalence of severe hypovitaminosis D in patients with persistent, nonspecific musculoskeltal pain. Mayo Clin Proc, 2003. **78**: p1463-1470.

225. Lewis, P.J., *Vitamin D deficiency may have role in chronic low back pain.* BMJ, 2005. **331** (7508): p109.

226. Hameed, K., Gibson, T., *A comparison of the prevalence of rheumatoid arthritis and other rheumatic diseases amongst Pakistanis living in England and Pakistan.* Br J Rheumatol, 1997. **36** (7): p781-5.

227. Helliwell, P., *et al.*, *Unexplained musculoskeletal pain in people of South Asian ethnic group referred to a rheumatology clinic — relationship to biochemical osteomalacia, persistance over time and response to treatment with calcium and vitamin D.* Clin Exp Rheumatol, 2006. **24** (4): p424-7.

228. Torrente de la Jara, G., Pecoud, A., Favrat, B., *Musculoskeletal pain in female asylum seekers with hypovitaminosis D3.* BMJ, 2004. **329**: p156-7.

229. MacGregor, D.M., White, M.I., *Sunburn in children — the Aberdeen experience.* Clin Exp Dermatol, 2001. **26** (2): p137-40.

230. Lamprecht, S., Lipkin, M., *Chemoprevention of colon cancer by calcium, vitamin D and folate: molecular mechanisms.* Nat Rev Cancer, 2003. **3**: p601-14.

231. Shapiro, J.A., *et al.*, *Diet and rheumatoid arthritis in women: a possible protective effect of fish consumption.* Epidemiology, 1996. **7** (3): p256-63.

232. Benito-Garcia, E., *et al.*, *Protein, iron, and meat consumption and risk for rheumatoid arthritis: a prospective cohort study.* Arthritis Res Ther, 2007. **9** (1): pR16.

233. Skoldstam, L., Hagfors, L., Johannson, G., *An experimental study of a Mediterranean diet intervention for patients with rheumatoid arthritis.* Ann Rheum Dis, 2003. **3**: p208-214.

234. McKellar, G., *et al.*, *A pilot study of a Mediterranean-type diet intervention in female patients with rheumatoid arthritis living in areas of social deprivation in Glasgow.* Ann Rheum Dis, 2007. **66** (9): p1239-43.

235. Merlino, L.A., *et al.*, *Vitamin D intake is inversely associated with rheumatoid arthritis: results from the Iowa Women's Health Study.* Arthritis Rheum, 2004. **50** (1): p72-7.

236. Costenbader, K.H., *et al.*, *Vitamin D intake and risks of systemic lupus erythematosus and rheumatoid arthritis in women.* Ann Rheum Dis, 2007.

237. Nielen, M.M., *et al.*, *Vitamin D deficiency does not increase the risk of rheumatoid arthritis: comment on the article by Merlino* et al. Arthritis Rheum, 2006. **54** (11): p3719-20.

238. Forman, J.P., *et al.*, *Vitamin D intake and risk of incident hypertension: results from three large prospective cohort studies.* Hypertension, 2005. **46** (4): p676-82.

239. Pattison, D.J., Harrison, R.A., Symmons, D.P., *The role of diet in susceptibility to rheumatoid arthritis: a systematic review.* J Rheumatol, 2004. **31** (7): p1310-9.

240. Sonnenberg, A., McCarty, D., Jacobsen, S., *Geographic variation of inflammatory bowel disease within the United States.* Gastroenterology, 1991. **100**: p143-9.

241. Stone, M.A., Mayberry, J.F., Baker, R., *Prevalence and management of inflammatory bowel disease: a cross-sectional study from central England.* Eur J Gastroenterol Hepatol, 2003. **15** (12): p1275-80.

242. Rubin, G.P., *et al.*, *Inflammatory bowel disease: epidemiology and management in an English general practice population.* Aliment Pharmacol Ther, 2000. **14** (12): p1553-9.

243. Kyle, J., *Crohn's disease in the North eastern and Northern Isles of Scotland: An epidemiological review.* Gastroenterology, 1992, **103**: p392-399.

244. Lindberg, E., *et al.*, *Inflammatory bowel disease in children and adolescents in Sweden.* J Ped Gastroenterol and Nutr, 2000. **30**: p259-64.

245. Berner, J., Kier, T., *Ulcerative colitis and Crohn's disease in the Faroe Islands 1964-83. A retropsective epidemiological survey.* Scand J Gastroenterol, 1986. **2**: p188-193.

246. Sawczenk, A., *et al.*, *Prospective survey of childhood inflammatory bowel disease in the British Isles.* Lancet, 2001. **357**: p1093-4.

247. Armitage, E., *et al.*, *Incidence of juvenile-onset Crohn's disease in Scotland: association with northern latitude and affluence.* Gastroenterology, 2004. **127** (4): p1051-7.

248. Barton, J., Ferguson, A., *Clinical features, morbidity and mortality of Scottish children with inflammatory bowel disease.* Q J Med, 1990. **75** (277): p423-39.

249. Loftus, E.J., *Clinical epidemiology of inflammatory bowel disease: incidence, prevalence, and environmental influences.* Gastroenterology, 2004. **126**: p1504-1517.

250. Siffledeen, J., *et al.*, *The frequency of vitamin D deficiency in adults.* Can J Gastroenterol, 2003.

17 (8): p473-8.

251. Lamb, E., *et al.*, *Metabolic bone disease is present at diagnosis in patients with inflammatory bowel disease.* Alimentary Pharmacology and Therapy, 2002. **16**: p1895-1902.

252. Tajika, M., *et al.*, *Risk factors for vitamin D deficiency in patients with Crohn's disease.* J Gastroenterol, 2004. **39** (6): p527-33.

253. Roth, D.E., *et al.*, *Association between vitamin D receptor gene polymorphisms and response to treatment of pulmonary tuberculosis.* J Infect Dis, 2004. **190** (5): p920-7.

254. Vogelsang, H., *et al.*, *Bone disease in vitamin D-deficient patients with Crohn's disease.* Dig Dis Sci, 1989. **34** (7): p1094-9.

255. Klaus, J., *et al.*, *High prevalence of osteoporotic vertebral fractures in patients with Crohn's disease.* Gut, 2002. **51**: p654-8.

256. Rang, E., Brooke, B., Hermon-Taylor, J., *Association of ulcerative colitis with multiple sclerosis.* Lancet, 1982. **2**: p555.

257. Mizuno, T.M., Makimura, H., Mobbs, C.V., *The physiological function of the agouti-related peptide gene: the control of weight and metabolic rate.* Ann Med, 2003. **35** (6): p425-33.

258. Millen, A., *et al.*, *Diet and melanoma in a case-control study.* Cancer Epidemiology Biomarkers Prevention, 2004. **13** (6): p1042-1051.

259. Kidder, L.S., *et al.*, *Skeletal effects of sodium fluoride during hypokinesia.* Bone Miner, 1990. **11** (3): p305-18.

260. Grant, W.B., Moan, J., Reichrath, J., *Comment on "the effects on human health from stratospheric ozone depletion and its interactions with climate change" by M. Norval, A. P. Cullen, F. R. de Gruijl, J. Longstreth, Y. Takizawa, R. M. Lucas, F. P. Noonan and J. C. van der Leun, Photochem. Photobiol. Sci., 2007, 6, 232.* Photochem Photobiol Sci, 2007. **6** (8): p912-5; discussion 916-8.

261. Ma, Y., *et al.*, *Identification and characterization of non-calcemic, tissue-selective, non-secosteroidal vitamin D receptor modulators.* J Clin Invest, 2006. **116** (4): p892-904.

262. Kong, J., *et al.*, *Novel role of the vitamin D receptor in maintaining the integrity of the intestinal Mucosal barrier.* Am J Physiol Gastrointest Liver Physiol, 2007.

263. Li, Y.C., *et al.*, *1,25-Dihydroxyvitamin D(3) is a negative endocrine regulator of the renin-angiotensin system.* J Clin Invest, 2002. **110** (2): p229-38.

264. Riou, J. P., *et al.*, *The association between melanoma, lymphoma, and other primary neoplasms.* Archives Surgery, 1995. **130**: p1056-1061.

265. Jantchou, P., Monnet, E., Carbonnel, F., [*Environmental risk factors in Crohn's disease and ulcerative colitis (excluding tobbacco and appendicectomy*]. Gastroenterol Clin Biol, 2006. **30** (6-7): p859-67.

266. ISAAC Steering committee. *Worldwide variation in the prevalence of symptoms of asthma, allergic rhinoconjunctivitis & atopic eczema: ISAAC.* Lancet, 1998. **351**: p1225-32.

267. Kaur, B., *et al.*, *Prevalence of asthma symptoms, diagnosis, and treatment in 12-14 year old children across Great Britain (international study of asthma in childhood, ISAAC, UK).* BMJ, 1998. **316**: p118-24.

268. Hill, J., Thomson, N., *The changing epidemiology of asthma.* Scot Med J, 1998. **43**: p67-9.

269. Weiss, S., Litonjua, A., *Maternal diet vs lack of exposure to sunlight as the cause of the epidemic of asthma, allergies and other autoimmune diseases.* Thorax, 2008. **62**: p746-748.

270. Upton, M.N., *et al.*, Intergenerational 20 year trends in the prevalence of asthma and hay fever in adults: the Midspan family study surveys of parents and offspring. BMJ, 2000. **321** (7253): p88-92.

271. Iversen, L., *et al.*, *Is living in a rural area good for your respiratory health? Results from a cross-sectional study in Scotland.* Chest, 2005. **128** (4): p2059-67.

272. Devereux, G., *et al.*, *Low maternal vitamin E intake during pregnancy is associated with asthma in 5-year-old children.* Am J Respir Crit Care Med, 2006. **174** (5): p499-507.

273. Willers, S.M., *et al.*, *Maternal food consumption during pregnancy and asthma, respiratory and atopic symptoms in 5-year-old children.* Thorax, 2007. **62** (9): p773-9.

274. Camargo, C.A., Jr., *et al.*, *Maternal intake of vitamin D during pregnancy and risk of recurrent wheeze in children at 3y of age.* Am J Clin Nutr, 2007. **85** (3): p788-95.

275. Devereux, G., *et al.*, *Maternal vitamin D intake during pregnancy and early childhood wheezing.* Am J Clin Nutr, 2007. **85** (3): p853-9.

275.1 Camargo, C.A., *Cord blood 25-hydroxyvitamin D levels and risk of childhood wheeze in New Zealand.* Abstract: American Thoracic Society Conference, Toronto, 2008.

276. Black, P.N., Scragg, R., *Relationship between serum 25-hydroxyvitamin D and pulmonary function in the*

third national health and nutrition examination survey. Chest, 2005. **128** (6): p3792-8.

277.   Burns, J., *Low levels of vitamin D in teens may affect lung function.*, in *American Thoracic Society* International Conference 2006, press release ATC: San Diego, USA.

278.   Schuemann, B., *et al.*, *Low serum vitamin D levels are associated with greater risks for severe exacerbations in childhood asthmatics.* in *Biomarkers for pediatric asthma and atopy.* American Thoracic Society. 2008. Toronto.

279.   Xystrakis, E., *et al.*, *Reversing the defective induction of IL-10-secreting regulatory cells in glucocorticoid-resistant asthma patients.* Journal of Clinical Investigation, 2005. **116** (1): p146-155.

280.   Sears, M., *et al.*, *Long-term relation between breastfeeding and development of atopy and asthma in children and young adults: a longitudinal study.* Lancet, 2002. **360**: p901-7.

281.   Oddy, W., *et al.*, *Association between breast feeding and asthma in 6 year old children: findings of a prospective birth cohort study.* BMJ, 1999. **319**: p815-19.

282.   Romieu, I., *et al.*, *Breastfeeding and asthma among Brazilian children.* J Asthma, 2000. **37**: p575-83.

283.   Wafula, E., *et al.*, *Effects of passive smoking and breast-feeding on childhood bronchial asthma.* East Afr Med J, 1999. **76**: p606-9.

284.   Kaplan, B., Mascie-Taylor, C., *Biosocial factors in the epidemiology of childhood asthma in a British national sample.* J Epidemiol Commun Health, 1985. **39**: p152-56.

285.   Wilson, A., *et al.*, *Relation of infant diet to childhood health: seven year follow up of cohort of children in Dundee infant feeding study.* BMJ, 1998. **316**: p21-25.

286.   Rottem, M., Shoenfeld, Y., *Asthma as a paradignmfor autoimmune disease.* Int Arch Allergy Immunol, 2003. **132** (3): p210-4.

287.   Stene, L., Nafstad, P., *Relations between occurrence of type 1 diabetes and asthma.* Lancet, 2001. **357**: p607-8.

288.   Douek, I., *et al.*, *Children with type 1 diabetes and their unaffected siblings have fewer symptoms of asthma.* Lancet, 1999. **353**: p1850.

289.   Wjst, M., Dold, S., *Genes, factor X and allergens. What causes allergic diseases?* Allergy, 1999. **54**: p757-9.

290.   Shaheen, S., *Vitamin D deficiency and the asthma epidemic.* Thorax, 2008. **63** (3): p293.

291.   Wjst, M., *The vitamin D slant on allergy.* Pediatr Allergy Immunol, 2006. **17**: p477-483.

292.   Gale, C., *et al.*, *Maternal vitamin D status during pregnancy and child outcomes.* European J Clin Nutr, 2008. **62**: p68-77.

293.   Hypponen, E., *et al.*, *Infant vitamin d supplementation and allergic conditions in adulthood: northern Finland birth cohort 1966.* Ann N Y Acad Sci, 2004. **1037**: p84-95.

294.   Tobias, J., Cooper, C., *PTH/PTHrP Activity and the programming of skeletal development* in utero. Journal of Bone and Mineral Research, 2004. **19** (2): p177-182.

295.   Landin, L., Nilsson, B., *Bone Mineral content in children with fractures.* Clin Orthop, 1983. **178**: p292-296.

296.   Jones, I., *et al.*, *Four-year gain in bone mineral in girls with and without past forearm fractures: A DXA study. Dual X-ray absorptiometry.* J Bone Miner Res, 2002. **17**: p1065-1072.

297.   Javaid, M., *et al.*, *Maternal vitamin D status during late pregnancy and accrual of childhood bone mineral.* J Bone Miner Res, 2003. **18**: pS1-S13.

298.   Manias, K., McCabe, D., Bishop, N., *Fractures and recurrent fractures in children; varying effects of environmental factors as well as bone size and mass.* Bone, 2006. **39** (3): p652-7.

299.   Mauck, K.F., Clarke, B.L., *Diagnosis, screening, prevention, and treatment of osteoporosis.* Mayo Clin Proc, 2006. **81** (5): p662-72.

300.   Williamson, S., Greene, S., *Prevention message is not getting through.* BMJ, 2007. **334**: p1288.

301.   Henderson, C., *et al.*, *Predictors of total body bone mineral density in non-corticosteroid-treated prepubertal children with juvenile rheumatoid arthritis.* Arthritis and Rheumatism, 1997. **40** (11): p1967-1975.

302.   Hollis, B., Wagner, C., *Nutritional vitamin D status during pregnancy: reasons for concern.* CMAJ, 2006. **174** (9): p1287-90.

303.   Hollis, B., Wagner, C., *Assessment of dietary vitamin D requirements during pregnancy and lactation.* American Journal of Clinical Nutrition, 2004. **79** (5): p717-726.

304.   Dunnigan, M., *et al.*, *Meat consumption reduces the risk of nutritional rickets and osteomalacia.* British Journal of Nutrition, 2005. **94**: p983-991.

305.   Dunnigan, M., *et al.*, *Late rickets and osteomalacia in the Pakistani community in Glasgow.* Scott Med J, 1962. **7**: p159-167.

306. Callaghan, A.L., *et al.*, *Incidence of symptomatic vitamin D deficiency.* Arch Dis Child, 2006. **91** (7): p606-7.

307. Mughal, M., *et al.*, *Florid rickets associated with prolonged breast-feeding without vitamin D supplementation.* BMJ, 1999. **318** (7175): p39-40.

308. Wharton, B., Bishop, N., *Rickets.* Lancet, 2003. **362** (9393): p1389-400.

309. Shaw, N., Pal, B., *Vitamin D deficiency in UK Asian families: activating a new concern.* Arch Dis Child, 2002. **86**: p147-9.

310. Dunnigan, M., *et al.*, *Policy for prevention of Asian rickets in Britain: a preliminary assessment of the Glasgow rickets campaign.* BMJ, 1981. **282**: p357-360.

311. Lunt, M., *et al.*, *Defining incident vertebral deformities in population studies: a comparison of morphometric criteria.* Osteoporos Int, 2002. **13** (10): p809-15.

312. van Staa, T.P., *et al.*, *A simple score for estimating the long-term risk of fracture in patients using oral glucocorticoids.* QJM, 2005. **98** (3): p191-8.

313. Prentice, A., *Diet, nutrition and the prevention of osteoporosis.* Public Health Nutr, 2004. **7** (1A): p227-43.

314. Van Schoor, N., *et al.*, *Vitamin D deficiency as a risk for osteoporotic fractures.* Bone, 2008. **42** (2): p260-6.

315. Roddam, A., *et al.*, *Association between Plasma 25-hydroxyvitamin D levels and fracture risk.* American Journal of Epidemiology, 2007. **166** (11): p1327-1336.

316. Schlesinger, N., *et al.*, *Acute Gouty Arthritis is Seasonal.* The Journal of Rheumatology, 1998. **25**: p342-4.

317. van Staa, T.P., *et al.*, *Public health impact of adverse bone effects of oral corticosteroids.* Br J Clin Pharmacol, 2001. **51** (6): p601-7.

318. Knowelden, J., Buhr, A., Dunbar, O., *Incidence of fractures in persons over 35 years of age.* A report to the MRC working party on fractures in the elderly. Br J Prev Soc Med, 1964. **18**: p130-141.

319. Ooms, M., *et al.*, *Prevention of bone loss by vitamin D supplementation in elderly women: a randomised double-blind trial.* Journal of Clinical Endocrinology and Metabolism, 1995. **80**: p1052-8.

320. Peacock, M., *Nutritional aspects of hip fractures.* Challenges of Modern Medicine, 1995. **7**: p213-222.

321. Chalmers, J., *Vitamin D deficiency in elderly people.* BMJ, 1991. **303** (6797): p314-5.

322. Diamond, T., *et al.*, *Hip fracture in elderly men: the importance of subclinical vitamin D deficiency and hypogonadism.* Medical Journal of Australia, 1998. **169**: p138-41.

323. LeBoff, M., *et al.*, *Dietary and lifestyle factors affecting Asian children living in England.* European Journal of Clinical Nutrition, 1999. **53**: p268-272.

324. Fisher, A., *et al.*, *Relationships between myocardial injury, all-cause mortality, vitamin D, PTH, and biochemical bone turnover markers in older patients with hip fractures.* Annals of Clinical and Laboratory Science, 2007. **37** (3): p222-232.

325. Dawson-Hughes, B., *et al.*, *Vitamin D Round Table discussion about optimal vitamin D for osteoporosis.* Proceedings of Round Table discussion, Lausanne, Switzerland, 2004.

326. Chapuy, M., *et al.*, *Vitamin D3 and calcium to prevent hip fractures in eldelry women.* New England Journal of Medicine, 1992. **327**: p1637-42.

327. Trivedi, D., Doll, R., Khaw, K., *Effect of four monthly oral vitamin D3 (cholecalciferol) supplementation on fractures and mortality in men and women living in the community: randomised double blind controlled trial.* British Medical Journal, 2003. **326**.

328. Bischoff-Ferrari, H., *et al.*, *Fracture prevention with vitamin D supplementation: a meta-analysis of randomised controlled trials.* JAMA, 2005. **293** (18): p2257-64.

329. Francis, R.M., *The vitamin D paradox.* Rheumatology (Oxford), 2007. **46** (12): p1749-50.

330. Bischoff-Ferrari, H.A., *et al.*, *Fracture prevention with vitamin D supplementation: a meta-analysis of randomized controlled trials.* JAMA, 2005. **293** (18): p2257-64.

331. Avenell, A., *et al.*, *Vitamin D and vitamin D analogues for preventing fractures associated with involutional and post-menopausal osteoporosis.* Cochrane Database Syst Rev, 2005. **3**: pCD000227.

332. Boonen, S., *et al.*, *Need for additional calcium to reduce the risk of hip fracture with vitamin D supplementation: evidence from a comparative meta-analysis of randomized controlled trials.* J Clin Endocrinol Metab, 2007. **92** (4): p1415-23.

333. Tang, B.M., *et al.*, *Use of calcium or calcium in combination with vitamin D supplementation to prevent fractures and bone loss in people aged 50 years and older: a meta-analysis.* Lancet, 2007. **370** (9588): p657-66.

334. Bischoff-Ferrari, H., *How to select the doses of vitamin D in the management of osteoporosis.* Osteoporosis International, 2007. **18**: p401-407.

335. Lips, P., *et al.*, *Vitamin D supplementation and fracture incidence in elderly persons. A randomized,*

placebo-controlled clinical trial. Ann Intern Med, 1996. **124** (4): p400-6.

336. Grant, A.M., *et al.*, *Oral vitamin D3 and calcium for secondary prevention of low-trauma fractures in elderly people (Randomised Evaluation of Calcium Or vitamin D, RECORD): a randomised placebo-controlled trial.* Lancet, 2005. **365** (9471): p1621-8.

337. Jackson, R.D., *et al.*, *Calcium plus vitamin D supplementation and the risk of fractures.* N Engl J Med, 2006. **354** (7): p669-83.

338. Lappe, J.M., *et al.*, *Calcium and vitamin D supplementation decreases incidence of stress fractures in female navy recruits.* J Bone and Mineral Research, 2008. **23**: p741-749.

339. Hathcock, J., *et al.*, *Risk assessment for vitamin D.* Am. J. Clinical Nutrition, 2007. **85** (1): p6-18.

340. Donaldson, L., *et al.*, *The epidemiology of fractures in England.* Journal of Epidemiology and Community Health, 2008. **62**: p174-180.

341. Riggs, B., L. Melton, L., *The worldwide problem of osteoporosis: Insights afforded by epidemiology.* Bone, 1995. **17 Supplement** (5): p505S-511S.

342. Arrott, S., *The economic cost of hip fracture in the UK. A paper commissioned by the Department of Trade and Industry.* 2000, York: Centre for Health Economics, University of York.

343. *National Service Framework for Older People.* 2001, Department of Health: London.

344. Skedros, J.G., Holyoak, J.D., Pitts, T.C., *Knowledge and opinions of orthopaedic surgeons concerning medical evaluation and treatment of patients with osteoporotic fracture.* J Bone Joint Surg Am, 2006. **88** (1): p18-24.

345. King, J., *Dental disease in the island of Lewis.* 1940, Medical Research Council: London.

346. East, B., *Mean annual hours of sunshine and the incidence of dental caries.* American Journal of Public Health, 1939. **29**: p777-780.

347. Brooke, R.C., *et al.*, *Discordance between facial wrinkling and the presence of basal cell carcinoma.* Arch Dermatol, 2001. **137** (6): p751-4.

348. Purvis, R., *et al.*, *Enamel hyoplasia of the teeth associated with neonatal tetany: manifestation of maternal vitamin deficiency.* Lancet, 1973. **2**: p811-814.

349. Skinner, H.G., *et al.*, *Vitamin D intake and the risk for pancreatic cancer in two cohort studies.* Cancer Epidemiol Biomarkers Prev, 2006. **15** (9): p1688-95.

350. Krall, E., *The periodontal-systemic connection: implications for treatment of patients with osteoporosis and periodontal disease.* Ann Periodontol, 2001. **6** (1): p209-13.

351. Inagaki, K., *et al.*, *Low metacarpal bone density, tooth loss, and periodontal disease in Japanese women.* J Dent Res, 2001. **80** (9): p1818-22.

352. Michaud, D., *et al.*, *Periodontal disease, tooth loss, and cancer risk in male health professionals: A prospective cohort study.* Lancet Oncology, 2008. **9**: p550-58.

353. Janssen, H., Samson, M., Verhaar, H., *Vitamin D deficiency, muscle function, and falls in elderly people.* Am J Clin Nutr, 2002. **76** (6): p1454-5 author reply 1455-6.

354. Pfeiffer, M., Begerow, B., Minne, H., *Vitamin D and muscle function.* Osteoporosis International, 2002. **13** (3): p187-94.

355. Bischoff, H.A., *et al.*, *Relationship between muscle strength and vitamin D metabolites: are there therapeutic possibilities in the elderly?* Z Rheumatol, 2000. **59 Suppl 1**: p39-41.

356. Ritz, E., Boland, R., Kreusser, W., *Effects of vitamin D and parathyroid hormone on muscle: potential role in uraemic myopathy.* American Journal of Clinical Nutrition, 1980. **33**: p1522-29.

357. Rimaniol, J., Authier, F., Chariot, P., *Muscle weakness in intensive care patients' initial manifestation of vitamin D deficiency.* Intensive Care Medicine, 1994. **20**: p591-2.

358. Bischoff, H.A., *et al.*, *Effects of vitamin D and calcium supplementation on falls: a randomized controlled trial.* J Bone Miner Res, 2003. **18** (2): p343-51.

359. Plotnikoff, G.A., *Vitamin D – the steroid hormone prescription for every patient.* Minn Med, 2003. **86** (1): p43-5.

360. Venning, G., *Recent developments in vitamin D deficiency and muscle weakness among elderly people.* BMJ, 2005. **330** (7490): p524-6.

361. Nellen, J., *et al.*, *Hypovitaminosis D in immigrant women slow to be diagnosed.* BMJ, 1996. **312**: p.570-2.

362. Rhein, H., *Vitamin D levels in a sample of 99 General Practice patients in Edinburgh.*, personal communication to O. Gillie, 2008: Edinburgh/London.

363. Maniadakis, N., Gray, A., *The economic burden of backpain in the UK.* Pain, 2000. **84**: p95-103.

364. Dukas, L., et al., *Alfacalcidol reduces the number of fallers in a community-dwelling elderly population with a minimum calcium intake of more than 500 mg daily.* J Am Geriatr Soc, 2004. **52** (2): p230-6.

365. Jeckson, C., et al., *The effect of cholecalciferol (vitamin D3) on the risk of fall and fracture: a meta-analysis.* Quarterly Journal of Medicine, 2007.

366. Wicherts, I.S., et al., *Vitamin D status predicts physical performance and its decline in older persons.* J Clin Endocrinol Metab, 2007. **92** (6): p2058-65.

367. Houston, D.K., et al., *Association between vitamin D status and physical performance: the In CHIANTI study.* J Gerontol A Biol Sci Med Sci, 2007. **62** (4): p440-6.

368. Hoogendijk, W., et al., *Depression is associated with decreased 25-hydroxyvitamin D and increased parathyroid hormone levels in older adults.* Arch Gen Psychiatry, 2008. **65** (5): p508-12.

369. El-Hajj Fuleihan, G., et al., *Effect of vitamin D replacement on musculoskeletal parameters in school children: a randomized controlled trial.* J Clin Endocrinol Metab, 2006. **91** (2): p405-12.

370. Chuck, A., Todd, J., Diffey, B., *Subliminal ultraviolet-B irradiation for the prevention of vitamin D deficiency in the elderly: a feasibility study.* Photodermatol Photoimmunol Photomed, 2001. **17** (4): p168-71.

371. Cannell, J., *Peak athletic performance and vitamin D.* The Vitamin D newsletter, 2007. March.

372. Lovell, G., *Vitamin D status of females in an elite gymnastics program.* Clin J Sport Med, 2008. **18** (2): p159-61.

373. *Nutrition and bone health: with particular reference to vitamin D. Report on Health and Social Subjects No 49.* UK Department of Health. 1998, Stationery Office.

374. Cannell, J., et al., *Diagnosis and treatment of vitamin D deficiency.* Expert Opin. Pharmacother., 2008. **9** (1): p1-12.

375. Parade, G., Otto, H., *Die beeinflussung der leistungsfahigkeit durch Hohensonnenbestrahlung.* Z Klin Med, 1940. **137**: p17-21.

376. Gorkin, Z.D., Dantsig, N.M., *[The current status and future perspectives of the use of ultraviolet rays in the prevention of light deficiency].* Vestn Akad Med Nauk SSSR, 1967. **22** (8): p58-62.

377. Willis, K., Peterson, N., Larson-Meyer, D., *Should we be concerned about the vitamin D status of athletes?* International Journal of Sport Nutrition and Exercise Metabolism, 2008. **18**: p204-224.

378. Hame, S., et al., *Fractures in the Collegiate athlete.* Am J Sports Med, 2004. **32** (2): p446-51.

379. Klesges, R., et al., *Changes in bone mineral content in male athletes: Mechanisms of action and intervention effects.* JAMA, 1996. 276: p. 226-230.

380. Chan, T., *Vitamin D deficiency and susceptibility to tuberculosis.* Calcified Tissue International, 2000. **66**: p476-478.

381. Bellamy, R., *Evidence of gene-environment interaction in development fo tuberculosis.* Lancet, 2000. **355** (9204): p588.

382. Arunabh, S., et al., *Body fat content and 25-hydroxyvitamin D levels in healthy women.* J Clin Endocrinol Metab, 2003. **88** (1): p157-61.

383. Gallerani, M., Manfredini, R., *Seasonal variation in herpes zoster infection.* Br J Dermatol, 2000. **142**: p560-1.

384. Rogan, M., et al., *Antimicrobial proteins and polypeptides in pulmonary innate defence.* Respiratory Research, 2006. **7**: p29.

385. Tse, S.L., et al., *Deficient dietary vitamin K intake among elderly nursing home residents in Hong Kong.* Asia Pac J Clin Nutr, 2002. **11** (1): 62-5.

386. Laaksi, I., et al., *An association of serum vitamin D concentrations <40 nmol/L with acute resiratory tract infection in young Finnish men.* American Journal of Clinical Nutrition, 2007. **86** (3): p714-717.

387. Yusuf, S., et al., *The relationship of meteorological conditions to the epidemic activity of respiratory syncitial virus.* Epidemiol Infect, 2007.

388. Douglas, A., Strachan, D., Maxwell, J., *Seasonality of tuberculosis: the reverse of other respiratory diseases in the UK.* Thorax, 1996. **51**: p944-6.

389. Douglas, A., Shaukat, A., Bakhshi, S., *Does vitamin D deficiency account for ethnic differences in tuberculosis seasonality in the UK?* Ethnicity and Health, 1998. **3** (4): p247-53.

390. Perez-Trallero, E., et al., *Vitamin D and Tuberculosis Incidence in Spain.* Am. J. Respir. Crit. Care Med., 2008. **177** (7): p798-9.

391. Chan, T., et al., *A study of calcium and vitamin D metabolism in Chinese patients with pulmonary tuberculosis.* Journal of Tropical Medicine and Hygiene, 1994. **97**: p26-30.

392. Davies, P., *A possible link between vitamin D deficiency and impaired host defence to Mycobacterium tuberculosis.* Tubercle, 1985. **66**: p301-306.

393. Nnoaham, K., Clarke, A., *Low serum vitamin D levels and tuberculosis: a systematic review and meta-analysis.* International Journal of Epidemiology, 2008. **37** (1): p113-119.

394. Hewison, M., *Vitamin D and innate immunity.* Current Opinion in Investigational Drugs, 2008. **9**.

395. Hobday, R., *The healing Sun – sunlight and health in the 21st Century.* 1999, London: Findhorn Press.

396. Dowling, G., Prosser-Thomas, E., *Treatment of lupus vulgaris with calciferol.* Lancet, 1946. **i**: p919-22.

397. Martineau, A.R., *et al., A single dose of vitamin D enhances immunity to mycobacteria.* Am J Respir Crit Care Med, 2007. **176** (2): p208-13.

398. Martineau, A.R., *et al., Vitamin D in the treatment of pulmonary tuberculosis.* J Steroid Biochem Mol Biol, 2007. **103** (3-5): p793-8.

399. Kurtzke, J.F., Heltberg, A., *Multiple sclerosis in the Faroe Islands: an epitome.* J Clin Epidemiol, 2001. **54** (1): p1-22.

400. Cook, S., *et al., Declining incidence of multiple sclerosis in the Orkney Islands.* Neurology 1985. **35**: p545-551.

401. Cook, S., *et al., Multiple sclerosis in the Shetland Islands: an update.* Acta Neurol. Scand., 1988. **77**: p148-151.

402. Kurtzke, J.F., *Epidemiologic evidence for multiple sclerosis as an infection.* Clin Microbiol Rev, 1993. **6** (4): p382-427.

403. Kurtzke, J.F., Gudmundsson, K.R., Bergmann, S., *Multiple sclerosis in Iceland: 1. Evidence of a postwar epidemic.* Neurology, 1982. **32** (2): p143-50.

404. Benedikz, J., Magnusson, H., Gudmundsson, G., *Multiple sclerosis in Iceland, with observations on the alleged epidemic in the Faroe Islands.* Annals of Neurology, 1994. **36, supp 2**: pS175-S179.

405. Poser, C., *et al., Analysis of the 'epidemic' of multiple sclerosis in the Faroe Islands.* Neuroepidemiology, 1988. **7**: p168-180.

406. Poser, C., Hibberd, P., *Analysis of the "epidemic" of multiple sclerosis in the Faroe islands II. Biostatistical aspects.* Neuroepidemiology, 1988. **7**: p181-189.

407. Poskanzer, D., *et al., Studies in the epidemiology of multiple sclerosis in the Orkney and Shetland Islands.* Neurology, 1976. **26, part 2**: p14-7.

408. Kinlen, L. Balkwill, A., *Infective cause of childhood leukaemia and wartime population mixing in Orkney and Shetland, UK.* Lancet, 2001. **357**: p858.

409. Kinlen, L.J., *Childhood leukaemia and non-Hodgkins lymphoma in young people living close to nuclear reprocessing sites.* Biomed Pharmacother, 1993. **47** (10): p429-34.

410. Kinlen, L.J., *et al., Rural population mixing and childhood leukaemia: effects of the North Sea oil industry in Scotland, including the area near Dounreay nuclear site.* BMJ, 1993. **306** (6880): p743-8.

411. Mangelsdorf, D., *et al., Dihydroxyvitamin D3-induced differentiation in a human promyelocytic leukaemia cell line (HL-60): receptor-mediated maturation to macrophage-like cells.* Journal of Cell Biology, 1984. **98**: p391-398.

412. Miyaura, C., *et al., 1,25-Dihydroxyvitamin D3 induces differentiation of human myeloid leukaemia cells.* Biochemical and Biophysical Research Communications, 1981. **102**: p917-943.

413. James, S., *et al., Leukaemia cell differentiation: Cellular and molecular interactions of retimoids and vitamin D.* 1999. **32** (1): p143-154.

414. Trump, D., *et al., Vitamin D compounds: clinical developments as cancer therapy and prevention agents.* Anticancer Res, 2006. **26** (4A): p2551-6.

415. Luong, Q., Koeffler, H., *Vitamin D compounds in leukaemia.* J Steroid Biochem Mol Biol, 2005. **97** (1-2): p195-202.

416. Buckley, J., *et al., Multiple sclerosis in mothers of children with acute lymphoblastic leukemia.* Leukemia, 1989. **3** (10): p736-739.

417. Cartwright, R., *et al., Acute myeloid leukemia in adults: a case-control study in Yorkshire.* Leukemia, 1988. **2**: p687-690.

418. Vieth, R., *The pharmacology of vitamin D, Including fortification strategies. Vitamin D – 2nd edition,* ed. P. Feldman, Glorieux. 2005: Elsevier, Academic Press.

419. Moan, J., *et al., Colon cancer: prognosis for different latitudes, age groups and seasons in Norway.* J Photochem Photobiol B, 2007. **89** (2-3): p148-55.

420. Maclean, C., *Island on the Edge of the World: The Story of St Kilda.* First published 1980: Canongate Classics, Edinburgh.

421. Cluness, A., *The Shetland Isles.* 1951, London: Hale

422. Department of Health for Scotland. Report of Committee on Scottish Health Services. 1936: Edinburgh.

423. Cathcart, E., Murray, A., Beveridge, J.K., An inquiry into the Diet of Families in the Highlands and Islands of Scotland., in Studies in Nutrition. 1940, Medical Research Council, HMSO: London.

424. Hargreaves, J., Changes in diet and dental health of children living in the Scottish Island of Lewis. Caries Res, 1972. **6**: p355-376.

425. Poskanzer, D., et al., Multiple sclerosis in Orkney and Shetland Islands II: The search for an exogenous aetiology. J Epidemiology and Community Health, 1980. **34**: p240-252.

426. Whichelow, M., Prevost, A., Dietary patterns and their associations with demographic, lifestyle and health variables in a random sample of British adults. Br J Nutr, 1996. **76** (1): p17-30.

427. Walker, J., An Economic History of the Hebrides and Highlands of Scotland. 1808, London.

428. World Cancer Research Fund/American Institute for Cancer Research. Food, Nutrition, Physical Activity and the Prevention of Cancer: a Global Perspective. 2007, AICR: Washington DC.

429. Marmot, M., Food, Nutrition, Physical Activity, and the Prevention of Cancer: a Global Perspective. 2007, World Cancer Research Fund, American Institute of Cancer Research: Washington, DC.

430. Feltbower, R., et al., International parallels in leukaemia and diabetes epidemiology. Arch Dis Child, 2004. **89**: p54-56.

431. Shah, A., Coleman, M.P., Increasing incidence of childhood leukaemia: a controversy re-examined. Br J Cancer, 2007. **97** (7): p1009-12.

432. Dreifaldt, A., Carlberg, M., Hardell, L., Increasing incidence rates of childhood malignant diseases in Sweden during the period 1960-1998. Eur J Cancer, 2004. **40** (9): p1351-60.

433. Coleman, M., et al., Trends in Cancer Incidence and Mortality. No 121., in IARC Scientific Publications. 1993, International Agency for Research in Cancer: Lyon.

434. Wertman, E., Zilber, N., Abramsky, O., An association between multiple sclerosis and type 1 diabetes. J Neurol, 1992. **239** (1): p43-5.

435. Marrosu, M., et al., Patients with multiple sclerosis and risk of type 1 diabetes mellitus in Sardinia, Italy: a cohort study. Lancet, 2002. **359** (9316): p1461-5.

436. Nielsen, N., et al., Type 1 diabetes and multiple sclerosis: a Danish population-based study. Arch Neurol, 2006. **63** (7): p1001-4.

437. Boscoe, F., Schmura, M., Solar ultraviolet-B exposure and cancer incidence and mortality in the United States, 1993-2002. BMC Cancer, 2006. **6**: p264.

438. Greaves, M., Childhood leukaemia. British Medical Journal, 2002. **324**: p283-287.

439. Wiemels, J., et al., Prenatal origin of acute lymphoblastic leukaemia in children. Lancet, 1999. **354**.

440. Greaves, M., Aetiology of acute leukaemia. Lancet, 1997. **349**: p344-9.

441. Atkinson, S.A., et al., Bone and mineral abnormalities in childhood acute lymphoblastic leukemia: influence of disease, drugs and nutrition. Int J Cancer Suppl, 1998. **11**: p35-9.

442. Feltbower, R.G., et al., Seasonality of birth for cancer in Northern England, UK. Paediatr Perinat Epidemiol, 2001. **15** (4): p338-45.

443. Ederer, F., et al., Birth-month and infant cancer mortality. Lancet, 1965. July **24**: p185-186.

444. Ross, J., et al., Seasonal variations in the diagnosis of childhood cancer in the United States. British Journal of Cancer, 1999. **81**: p549-553.

445. Sorensen, H.T., et al., Seasonal variation in month of birth and diagnosis of early childhood acute lymphoblastic leukemia. JAMA, 2001. **285** (2): p168-9.

446. Philipps, A., Philips, J., Poster: Seasonal variation in month of birth of children diagnosed with acute lymphoblastic leukaemia and a possible relationship with light at night., in Childhood Leukaemia. Incidence, causal mechanisms and prevention. 2004: London.

447. Higgins, C.D., et al., Season of birth and diagnosis of children with leukaemia: an analysis of over 15,000 UK cases occurring from 1953-95. Br J Cancer, 2001. **84** (3): p406-12.

448. Meltzer, A.A., Annegers, J.F., Spitz, M.R., Month-of-birth and incidence of acute lymphoblastic leukemia in children. Leuk Lymphoma, 1996. **23** (1-2): p85-92.

449. Dalberg, J., et al., Colorectal cancer in the Faroe Islands – a setting for the study of the role of diet. J Epidemiol Biostat, 1999. **4** (1): p316.

450. Giovannucci, E., The epidemiology of vitamin D and colorectal cancer: recent findings. Curr Opin Gastroenterol, 2006. **22** (1): p24-9.

451. Giovannucci, E., Calcium plus vitamin D and the risk of colorectal cancer. N Engl J Med, 2006.

354 (21): p2287-8; author reply 2287-8.

452. Giovannucci, E., *Commentary: vitamin D and colorectal cancer—twenty-five years later.* Int J Epidemiol, 2006. **35** (2): p222-4.

453. Garland, C.F., *et al., The role of vitamin D in cancer prevention.* Am J Public Health, 2006. **96** (2): p252-61.

454. Hall, M., *et al.,* A 22-year prospective study of fish, n-3 fatty acid intake, and colorectal cancer risk in men. Cancer Epidemiology, Biomarkers & Prevention, 2008. **17**: p1136-43.

455. Berner, J., Kiaer, T., *Ulcerative colitis and Crohn's disease on the Faroe Islands 1964-83. A retrospective epidemiological survey.* Scand J Gastroenterol., 1986. **21** (2): p188-92.

456. Boucher, B., *Evidence of deficiency and insufficiency of vitamin D in the UK: National Diet and Nutrition Survey (NDNS) data. 1994-2004.* in *Sunlight, Vitamin D and Health. Report of a conference held at the House of Commons in November 2005.* Health Research Forum Occasional Reports, 2005. **2**: 53-56.

457. Gillie, O., *Sunlight Robbery: Health Benefits of sunlight are denied by current public health policy in the UK.* Health Research Forum Occasional Reports, 2004. **1**: p1-42.

458. Holick, M.F., M. Jenkins, M., *The UV Advantage.* 2003, USA: ibooks.

459. Gillie, O., *Sunbathing is needed for optimum health in the British Isles.* British Medical Journal, 2005. **331**: p. rapid response to editorial by Brian Diffey p3-4.

460. Sinclair, C., *Vitamin D – An Emerging Issue in Skin Cancer Control. Implications for Public Health Practice Based on the Australian Experience.* Recent Results in Cancer Research, 2007. **174**.

461. Samanek, A., *et al., Estimates of beneficial and harmful sun exposure times during the year for major Australian population centres.* MJA, 2006. **184** (7): p338-341.

462. Janda, M., *et al., Sun protection messages, vitamin D and skin cancer: out of the frying pan and into the fire?* Med J Aust, 2007. **186** (2): p52-53.

463. Lucas, R.M., *et al., Estimating the global disease burden due to ultraviolet radiation exposure.* Int J Epidemiol, 2008.

464. Gandini, S., *et al., Meta-analysis of risk factors for cutaneous melanoma: II Sun exposure.* European Journal of Cancer, 2005. **41**: p45-60.

465. Lucas, R.M., Ponsonby, A.L., *Considering the potential benefits as well as adverse effects of sun exposure: can all the potential benefits be provided by oral vitamin D supplementation?* Prog Biophys Mol Biol, 2006. **92** (1): p140-9.

466. Nickkho-Amiry, M., *et al., Maternal vitamin D status and breast milk concentrations of calcium and phosphorous.* Archives Disease in Childhood, 2008. **93**: p179.

467. Felton, D., Stone, W., *Osteomalacia in Asian immigrants during pregnancy.* British Medical Journal, 1966. **1**: p1521-1522.

468. Wagner, C., *et al., High-Dose Vitamin D3 Supplementation in a Cohort of Breastfeeding Mothers and Their Infants: A 6-Month Follow-Up Pilot Study.* Breastfeeding Medicine, 2006. **1**: p57-68.

469. Boucher, B., *Evidence of deficiency and insufficiency of vitamin D in the UK.* Health Research Forum Occassional Reports, 2006. B: p53-56.

470. DHSS, *Safe upper levels for vitamins and minerals.* Report of the expert group on vitamins and minerals., 2002: 133-140.

471. *Standing Committee on the Scientific Evaluation of Dietary Reference Intakes.* 1997: National Academy Press. USA.

472. *Health and Consumer Protectorate General. Opinion of the Scientific Committee on Food on the Tolerable Upper Intake Level of Vitamin D.* 2002, European Commission. .

473. Barger-Lux, M., Heaney, R., *Effects of above average summer sun exposure on serum 25-hydroxy-vitamin D and calcium absorption.* J Clin Endocrinol Metab, 2002. **87** (11): p4952-4956.

474. Heaney, R., *et al., Human serum 25-hydroxycholecalciferol response to extended oral dosing with cholecalciferol.* Am J Clin Nutr, 2003. **77** (1): p204-210.

475. Sharma, O., *Hypercalcemia in granulomatous disorders: a clinical review.* Current opinion in Pulmonary Medicine, 2000. **6**: p442-447.

476. Trang, H.M., *et al., Evidence that vitamin D3 increases serum 25-hydroxyvitamin D more efficiently than does vitamin D2.* Am J Clin Nutr, 1998. **68** (4): p854-8.

477. Holick, M., *et al., Vitamin D2 is as effective as vitamin D3 in maintaining circulating concentrations of 25-hydroxyvitamin D.* J Clin Endocrinol Metab., 2008: p. Dec 18 [Epub ahead of print].

478. Gillie, O., Mercer, D., *The Sunday Times book of body maintenance.* 1978, London: Michael Joseph.

479. Robsahm, T., *et al., Vitamin D3 from sunlight may improve the prognosis of breast colon and prostate cancer.* Cancer Causes and Control, 2004. **15**.

480. Berwick, M., *et al., Sun exposure and mortality from melanoma.* Journal of the National Cancer Institute, 2005. **97** (3).

481. Moan, J., *et al., Addressing the health benefits and risks, involving vitamin D or skin cancer, of increased sun exposure.* Proceedings of the National Academy of Sciences, 2008. **105**: p668-73.

482. Moan, J., *et al., Addressing the health benefits and risks, involving vitamin D or skin cancer, of increased sun exposure.* Proc Natl Acad Sci U S A, 2008. **105** (2): p668-73.

483. Gillie, O., *A new health policy for sunlight and vitamin D.* Health Research Forum Occasional Reports, 2005. **2**: p62-70.

484. Gillie, O., *A new government policy is needed for sunlight and vitamin D.* British Journal of Dermatology, 2005. **154**: p1052-61.

485. Gillie, O., *On the sunny side of the street,* in *The Guardian.* 2007: London. p. letters page.

486. Gillie, O., *Sunbathing comes out from under a cloud,* in *The Sunday Telegraph.* 2008. p. Comment section.

487. Moan, J., Dahlback, A., Setlow, R., *Epidemiological support for an hypothesis for melanoma induction indicating a role for UVA radiation.* Photochem Photobiol., 1999. **70** (2): p243-7.

488. Mowbray, M., Stockton, D., Doherty, V., *Changes in the site distribution of malignant melanoma in South East Scotland (1979-2002).* British Journal of Cancer, 2007. **96**: p832-835.

489. Dixon, K., *et al., In vivo relevance for photoprotection by the vitamin D rapid response pathway.* J Steroid Biochem. Mol. Biol., 2007: p. doi:10.10916/j.jsbmb.2006.11.016.

490. Webb, A.R., Engelson, O., *Calculated ultraviolet exposure levels for a healthy vitamin D status.* Photochem Photobiol. , 2006. **82** (6): p1697-703.

491. Hollis, B., *Circulating 25-hydroxyvitamin D levels indicative of vitamin sufficiency: implications for establishing a new effective dietary intake recommendation for vitamin D.* J Nutr, 2005. **135**: p317-322.

492. Webb, A., Engelsen, O., *Ultraviolet exposure scenarios: risks of erythema from recommendations on cutaneous vitamin D synthesis.* Adv Exp Med Biol 1 Jan 2008 **624**: p72-83.

493. Adams, J.S., *et al., Vitamin-D synthesis and metabolism after ultraviolet irradiation of normal and vitamin-D-deficient subjects.* N Engl J Med, 1982. **306** (12): p722-5.

494. Autier, P., *et al., Sunbed use and risk of melanoma: results from a large multicentric European study* in *XVIII International Pigment Cell Conference.* 2002: Egmond, Netherlands. p9-13 September 2002.

495. Porojnicu, A., *et al., Sun beds and cod liver oil as vitamin D sources.* Photobiology in press, 2008.

496. Giovannucci, E., *et al., Prospective study of predictors of vitamin D status and cancer incidence and mortality in men.* J Natl Cancer Inst, 2006. **98** (7): p451-9.

497. Berk, M., *et al., Vitamin D deficiency may play a role in depression.* Med Hypotheses, 2007. **69** (6): p1316-9.

498. Reinhold Vieth , S.K., Hul, A., Walfish, P.G., *Randomized comparison of the effects of the vitamin D3 adequate intake versus 100 mcg (4000 IU) per day on biochemical responses and the wellbeing of patients.* Nutrition Journal 2004. **3** (8).

499. Armstrong, D.J., *et al., Vitamin D deficiency is associated with anxiety and depression in fibromyalgia.* Clin Rheumatol, 2007. **26** (4): p551-4.

500. de Gruijl, F., *et al., Wavelength dependence of skin cancer induction by ultraviolet irradiation of albino hairless mice.* Cancer Res, 1993. **53**: p53-60.

501. Moan, J.,Dahlback, A., Setlow, R., *Epidemiological support for an hypothesis for melanoma induction indicating a role for UVA radiation.* Photochem. Photobiol., 1999. **70**: p243-247.

502. Garland, C.F., Garland, F.C., Gorham, E.D., *Epidemiologic evidence for different roles of ultraviolet A and B radiation in melanoma mortality rates.* Ann Epidemiol, 2003. **13** (6): p395-404.

503. Scotto, J., *et al., Non-melanoma skin cancer.* Cancer Epidemiology and Prevention (2nd edition), ed. D. Schottenfeld and J.J. Fraumeni. 1996, New York, USA: Oxford University Press. 1313-1330.

504. Lim, E.C., Terasaki, P.I., *Outcome of renal transplantation in different primary diseases.* Clin Transpl, 1991: p293-303.

505. Joseph, J., *The Gene Illusion – Genetic work in psychiatry and psychology under the microscope.* 2004, New York: Algora Publishing.

506. Gillie, O., *Sunlight, Vitamin D and Health.* 2006, London: Health Research Forum.

507. Gillie, O., *A new government policy is needed for sunlight and vitamin D.* British Journal of Dermatology 2006: p1052-1061.

Index